YOUR BABY'S CRY FOR HELP

Understanding and Helping Babies
Who Cry Excessively

Peter Zealley ND, DO, BCST

Copyright © 2014 by Peter Zealley, all rights reserved.

Peter Zealley has asserted his right under the Copyright, Designs and Patents Act 1988 to be identified as the author of this work.

No part of this book may be used or reproduced, stored in a retrieval system, or transmitted in any form or by any means, electronic, mechanical, photocopying, recording, scanning, or otherwise, except as permitted by the Copyright, Designs and Patents Act 1988, without either the prior written permission of the Author.

This book is sold subject to the condition that it shall not, by way of trade or otherwise, be lent, resold, hired out, or otherwise circulated without the author's prior consent in any form of binding or cover other than that in which it is published and without a similar condition, including this condition, being imposed on the subsequent purchaser.

Limit of Liability/Disclaimer of Warranty: While the Author has used his best efforts in preparing this book, he makes no representations or warranties with respect to the accuracy or completeness of the contents of this book and specifically disclaim any implied warranties of merchantability or fitness for a particular purpose. Nothing within the book should be taken as medical advice. The suggestions and strategies contained herein may not be suitable for your situation. If in doubt, you are advised to consult a qualified medical practitioner. The Author shall not be liable for any loss of profit or any other commercial damages, including but not limited to special, incidental, consequential, or other damages.

Author services by Pedernales Publishing, LLC

Interior illustrations by Edward Zealley

Author's photograph by Wendy Brooking

British Library Cataloguing in Publication Data

A catalogue record for this book is available from the British Library.

Paperback edition   ISBN 978-1-499106-37-4

DEDICATION

I dedicate this book to all those young souls who have passed through my hands over the years. I trust they have benefited as much from me as I have learnt from each and every one of them.

CONTENTS

DEDICATION iii

ACKNOWLEDGEMENTS ix

INTRODUCTION xi

1. YOUR BABY HAS ARRIVED! 1
   - TAKING STOCK 1
   - WHY BABIES CRY 6
   - YOUR BABY 11
   - WHEN YOUR BABY WON'T STOP CRYING 18

2. WHY SOME BABIES CRY EXCESSIVELY OR SCREAM 23
   - THEY ARE STILL EXPERIENCING THE EFFECTS OF THEIR BIRTH 24
   - THEY ARE IN PAIN 30
   - ILLNESS 37
   - SENSORY PROCESSING ISSUES 41

3. HOW THE EFFECTS OF BIRTH CAN CAUSE YOUR BABY TO CRY 47
   - SOME USEFUL PHYSIOLOGY 47
   - MECHANICAL STRAIN ISSUES ARISING DURING THE BIRTH PROCESS 55

THE STRESSED BABY 64

THE TRAUMATISED BABY 70

4. HOW YOUR BABY EMERGED INTO THE WORLD 77

NATURAL DELIVERY 77

INTERVENTIONS 83

THE PREMATURE BABY 88

SOME POSTNATAL ISSUES 95

5. HOW YOUR BABY CAN BE HELPED 101

WHAT IS CRANIAL THERAPY? 102

CRANIAL THERAPY, ANATOMY IN MOTION 107

HOW CRANIAL THERAPY WORKS 113

WHEN CRANIAL THERAPY FAILS TO HELP 121

6. TAKING YOUR BABY TO A CRANIAL THERAPIST .. 126

PREPARING FOR AN APPOINTMENT 127

ASSESSING YOUR BABY 132

THIS IS WHAT HAPPENS DURING A TREATMENT .. 140

WHAT TO EXPECT AFTER A TREATMENT 147

7. ADAPTATION TO BIRTH 155

LIFE IS OFTEN ABOUT ADAPTATION 156

ADAPTATION IN BABIES 161

ADAPTATIONS IN CHILDREN 167

- ADAPTATION IN ADULTS AND MOVING INTO PRESENT TIME 173
- YOUR NEXT STEP 182
  - THE BOOK REVIEW 182
  - YOUR NEXT STEP 184
  - PROFESSIONAL ASSOCIATIONS 188
  - THE ROLE FOR CRANIAL THERAPY 189
- ABOUT PETER ZEALLEY 191

ACKNOWLEDGEMENTS

Firstly, I wish to acknowledge Kevin Bermingham of www.kevinbermingham.com and Helen Turier of www.helenturier.com. Without their structured approach and mentoring programme this book would never have manifested. It is a 90-day book.

I acknowledge Michael Kern and the Craniosacral Therapy Educational Trust (CTET, www.cranio.co.uk) for guiding me in refining my understanding and practice of craniosacral therapy.

My book chapter and complete book reviewers completed an excellent job and in such a short space of time. I extend my thanks to: craniosacral therapist Duncan MacPherson of www.duncan-cst.com, active birth teacher Karin Walters of www.birthwise.net, intuitive life coach Dee Brodie of www.deebrodie.com, acupuncturist and zero-balancer Richard Walters, good friend Lorna Cowdrey, my brother John Zealley and participating parents Alex Mitchel and Margo Greenwood.

I thank photographer Wendy Brooking for my back cover photo, my son Edward Zealley for his medical illustrations (commissions taken) and his book review, my son Matthew for his IT input, Emma and Dylan for their story and finally, my wife Liz for being so accepting of me spending most evenings and weekends writing in the back room during the 90-day programme.

INTRODUCTION

This book is about very unsettled babies. If you are a mother, or parent and you are trying to cope with your baby, who cries excessively or screams, and no one understands why, yet you instinctively know that something must be upsetting them, this book is for you. Crying is a communication, your baby's cry for help.

I am a father of three children and also a grandfather. As a graduate osteopath and craniosacral therapist, I have over 20 years of hands-on experience working with and helping babies and children. During my career I have gained invaluable insight and understanding into why babies cry excessively, or scream and it is this knowledge that I will share with you.

The knowledge contained within these pages is based in the medical sciences of anatomy and physiology.

Understanding how the human body responds in situations of strain, stress and trauma explains many of the symptom patterns present in babies, children and adults. It also provides the key to enable you to understand why your own baby cries excessively, or screams and how he/she can be helped.

By reading this book, you will understand what you have not been told so far, that your baby's birth or postnatal experience may still be affecting them now and causing them to cry excessively or scream. I will explain how different symptom patterns and behaviours arise and give you sufficient understanding of the theory and practice of craniosacral therapy and cranial osteopathy to enable you to decide if trying either of these two related treatment approaches is appropriate for you and your baby.

A trained therapist is able to use their sense of touch to assess and understand your baby. Your baby's past experiences are memories held within their body. It is this same gentle touch that is used to support your baby and to help them recover. If, as a result, your baby becomes content now, not only will he/she begin to enjoy their life more, but your own life and that of your family will transform too.

This book is primarily written for mothers. If you are a father or a health professional, you may find that

INTRODUCTION

the subject matter of the book begins in earnest with Chapter Two although you will still benefit from reading Chapter One. The case studies shared are true. With the exception of Dylan, the clients have had their names changed and sometimes their sex. In order to make the book personal to you and your baby both male and female pronouns are used together.

Peter. E. Zealley.

Peter Zealley ND, DO, BCST

Chapter 1.
YOUR BABY HAS ARRIVED!

The intention of this chapter is to create a space for you to reflect on yourself and your baby and what you have experienced together. It also considers baby crying as a form of communication: your baby's cry for help.

TAKING STOCK

HOW ARE YOU NOW?
Take a moment, settle into your body, draw in a deep breath, now breathe out slowly and ask yourself the question, 'How am I doing right now?' Whatever your answer, there is no need to change anything; this is just a reality check. How you are right now is how it is and this is important for you to recognise. You may be

just fine but more likely you are over-tired, exhausted, worn out, stressed, in pain, just coping, failing to cope, wondering what's going on and when you are going to get a break. Any or all of this is normal for a mother with a young baby.

How you are right now may depend on several factors:

- what your experience of giving birth was like
- whether you have recovered sufficiently from the events of the birth
- whether you had surgery or sustained any injuries and if so, how well you are healing
- the level of support you have
- how your baby is
- the relationship you have with your baby

The chances are that you have not fully recovered from your birth experience and being a mum with a young baby is presenting you with more challenges than you anticipated.

YOUR BIRTH EXPERIENCE
As a mother, particularly if you are a first-time mother, your birthing experience may not have been anything like you expected. Yet, how could it have been, when you never knew what was going to happen next? Births regularly do not go according to plan and are

often longer, more exhausting and far more painful than anything you might have imagined. Furthermore, interventions and complications are sometimes not anticipated in a birth plan, unless you have had an elective caesarean. Giving birth can be a difficult and stressful experience as well as a joyous one.

You may have planned a home birth but ended up in hospital. Perhaps you planned a natural birth, but ended up with a forceps delivery or a caesarean section. You may have had to resort to pain relief, or had an epidural.

If you had given birth before, you already knew what to expect, so your preparation was likely to have been different. This time around you may have been more in tune with your body and its natural instincts and trusted that you had the strength and support to follow through the natural process of birth. On the other hand, there are times when a second birth is more difficult or traumatic than the first because of health issues, the positioning of the baby or other unforeseen complications.

RECUPERATION
The main challenge that you face after giving birth is that unless you are fortunate in having a contented baby, you have little or no time for rest and recuperation. Immediately you are home, you will be thrown into

a life of having to meet your baby's needs (and often the needs of others around you too).

Recuperation is important because if you do not have time to adequately recover and heal from giving birth, you are more likely to live and survive on your stress response. This means you are constantly on the alert and therefore liable to becoming exhausted and overwhelmed. If you have had surgery, some time for recuperation is vital. Failing to recover both physically and mentally from your birth experience is one factor indicated in the development of postnatal depression.

ENVIRONMENT AND SUPPORT
Following the birth, your health and the health of your baby are not just determined by what you both experienced during the birth process and how well you are recovering, but also by your environment and the amount of personal support available to you.

Your environment includes the place and area where you live, the circumstances of your life, who you share it with and how conducive this is to your well-being and that of your baby. It is amazing how many mothers move house or accommodation during the later stages of pregnancy or soon after birth. This may be to do with a desire to create a safer and more nurturing environment to bring up their child as well as to have more space. Sometimes it seems as if the baby is influencing where their family need to live.

Support is also very important for you as a mother. Being able to share the trials, tribulations, difficulties and excitements of having a baby makes life easier and more rewarding. Support comes from people who can be there for you. This could be someone you share your life with or live with, or other children you may already have, particularly if they are old enough to take on some responsibility. Having a circle of close friends or extended family members you can trust and turn to gives you more options for talking and for help with your baby, especially when you are in need.

Having good medical support is also necessary. It is important that you are heard – no one knows more about your baby than you, the mother.

If you are well supported, you have more to give your baby. Having little or no support is not ideal, but it is surprising how your support network can unexpectedly change for the better where your baby is concerned. You now have the opportunity to join mother and baby groups and the possibility of developing new friendships with other mothers. Health services offer support to new mothers too.

Ideally your baby's father is a good source of support. This depends on the quality of your relationship, how paternal he is, how he coped with the birth experience and how much paternity leave he is able to take if he is working. Fathers present at a traumatic birth can be deeply shocked at what they witness and this may in turn affect their ability to cope later too, particularly if your baby cries and screams a lot.

WHY BABIES CRY

CRYING IS COMMUNICATION
Unlike other mammals, which are able to stand up and run for survival within hours of their birth, human babies are totally dependent on their parents for everything from the start. For this reason a developing baby's brain is programmed with primitive reflexes, which make him/her perform certain survival tasks automatically. These reflexes include the sucking reflex, otherwise they would not know how to feed; the rooting reflex, where the baby automatically searches for a nipple to suck; the orientation reflex, which enables the baby to turn his/her neck to follow sound; and the grab reflex, which enables a baby to hold onto a finger and be lifted up by it. Crying is a reflex too that happens as a need arises.

Babies cry, this is normal and healthy. Crying is how your baby communicates to you as their parent; it is their voice. It is the only means of expression a young baby has. A young baby does not choose to cry, it happens automatically. His/her nervous system is programmed to do this; it is a reflex. The only way your baby can get your attention and let you know that they have a need, or that something is not right, is by opening his/her mouth and crying, or, if necessary, screaming. Crying usually stops when their needs are met. If your baby continues to cry, cries excessively, inconsolably, or screams, it is a communication that something is still not right: babies cry for a reason.

Some babies do not cry. If your baby does not cry you may think you have a really peaceful baby. This may be true. Your baby is content in him/herself and his/her body and you may be sensitive to meeting their needs, even before he/she needs to cry. However, in some babies the opposite is true. Sometimes when a baby is very quiet it can be a sign that he/she is traumatised from their birth. Such babies may also show signs of being not very responsive – they may make poor eye contact and their body may lack tone. A quiet but traumatised baby may become very vocal several weeks after birth, when their body begins to realise what they have been through during the birth itself. Such babies may also develop digestive problems and sleep issues.

As your baby continues to grow, he/she develops more complex ways to express their needs and how they are, ultimately forming language. Initially babies begin to make a wider range of sounds and facial expressions and also become able to express feelings of contentment and happiness by smiling and laughing. With time it becomes easier for you to understand your baby's communications, his/her needs, difficulties and joy. You will recognise when they are really enjoying being alive and when they need help and what this help needs to be. Crying may then occur only if he/she is in pain, ill, or upset, just like children and adults.

RECOGNISING DIFFERENT TYPES OF CRY

As you get to know your baby, especially if you are a first-time parent, you will begin to recognise different types of cry. Not all crying is the same. The tone and intensity of crying varies, as do the feelings that are expressed with it. Recognising different cries can help you to understand your baby and his/her needs and indicate how you can best meet them. Some common cries you may recognise are:

- the 'I am hungry' cry
- the 'tired' cry
- the 'I am feeling sorry for myself' cry
- the 'fed up and bored' cry
- the 'I want to be picked up' cry

- the 'I want to be changed' cry
- the 'angry' cry
- the 'drama queen' cry (exaggerated crying)

A very intense cry becomes a scream, and may indicate that your baby is in pain, or he/she is totally overwhelmed. Many babies become quickly overwhelmed by life outside the womb, especially when too much is going on around them: young babies prefer a simple life.

YOUR BABY'S NEEDS
Your baby will cry and sometimes scream when he/she has a need, which they want you to meet. Their hope is that you will hear them, understand what their need is and then respond to it. In normal circumstances, when your baby's need is met, he/she stops crying. Your baby's basic needs are:

- to feel safe
- to be fed
- to be warm
- to be clean
- to be held
- to sleep
- to receive attention
- to be seen for who they are, which is being loved

As you get to know your baby and you meet and anticipate his/her needs, he/she should begin to settle over the first two to three months and there should be no persistent crying or screaming.

THEY LET YOU KNOW WHEN SOMETHING IS WRONG
Babies are aware of what goes on, both inside their body and around them, even though they may not consciously know this. Like all living species, human beings have evolved over millions of years to survive and thrive and so our primitive nervous system is programmed in the womb to react to anything which is a potential threat, even as a newborn.

Your baby will automatically react to anything that causes him/her discomfort, or pain and to any situation that threatens them. The normal reflex action to pain or threat is to cry, sometimes severely, or to scream. Experiences your baby may perceive and react to by crying or screaming include:

- feeling unsafe
- being on his/her own for too long
- not knowing what is going on
- being overwhelmed
- being over-tired
- being bored
- being too hot or cold

- being in discomfort or pain
- being ill

Feeling safe is our primary need as a baby, as a child and as adults. We build our life around creating safety. For this reason young babies are rarely happy to be left alone for long and so, for example, trying to get them to sleep in their own bedroom immediately after birth may not work.

YOUR BABY

HOW IS YOUR BABY?
For a moment, pause for thought and ask yourself, 'How is my baby doing right now? Is he/she OK, have you got concerns about them, or are they struggling?

If they are doing OK, they may still be hard work but be feeding well, putting on weight, can be put down, are getting enough sleep day and night, and cry only when they have a need. They settle once their needs are met; they are content.

If you are concerned about them, your baby may be having feeding issues, have episodes of crying, some difficulty getting off to sleep and frequently wake, have trouble bringing up wind or appear to have some abdominal discomfort and often need to be picked up and carried. Your baby may also have enough good periods to enable you to cope.

If your baby is never OK, then he/she is struggling. A baby who struggles may:

- cry frequently, excessively or inconsolably
- scream for hours, as if in pain
- arch his/her spine and go rigid, or draw their legs up
- be constantly alert and fight to get to sleep
- be restless, waking every hour and crying at night and not napping during the daytime
- be impossible to put down
- be sad and unhappy; grumpy

If your baby is struggling, it is normal for you as a parent to struggle to cope with them. You may not understand why they are like this.

When you are a first-time mum, you have nothing to compare your experiences with, so if your baby is unsettled and cries a lot, you may assume all babies are like this, that this is normal and that you have to cope somehow. However, when you compare your baby with your friends' babies, you may realise that theirs are much more content than your own. If you already have one child, or more, and your first children were quite settled, you will quickly realise if your new baby is behaving differently and in a way that concerns you. Either way, you may instinctively know when something is just not right.

YOUR BABY'S BIRTH
Have you ever thought what it was like for your baby being born? What was the experience of birth from his/her point of view? Although you were both there together, involved in the same birth process, you had different perspectives. They were inside of you coming out; you were around them, helping them out. For that reason your baby's birth experience and how he/she coped with it may have been very different to your own.

If your experience of the birth was that it was a straightforward natural delivery, your baby may still have found it a big endurance test, got stressed and struggled to cope. If the birth was a very long, traumatic experience for you and with intervention, your baby may have been traumatised too, or, they may have coped well – some babies thrive on stress. You may have been OK with a caesarean section, yet your baby may have been shocked by it. There are many permutations.

How well your baby coped with his/her birth is determined by what happened, how long it took, what occurred afterwards and the resilience of their character.

What makes birth so different from other events in life is that it is a process that takes time. Most accidents and injuries, even severe ones like car crashes and falls, occur without warning and are over within seconds. Birth takes time, frequently many hours and sometimes days. Also, you had time for preparation because you knew beforehand that something was going to happen sometime soon, often with an exact date. Because birth takes time, your baby's body has to constantly react to and adjust to each stage of labour and delivery. There may come a point when the birth process becomes too much too bear. Your baby may react to this by becoming stressed or overwhelmed.

You and your baby may have to dig deep to find the resources to cope with birth and to recover from it. Babies rarely just emerge from their mother's womb and carry on as if nothing has happened. There is a relationship between what a baby experiences during the birth process, how completely he/she gets over it and how settled they are now.

ABOUT BABIES
Who your baby is as an individual, their personality, is set at conception. From that moment on they can never become anyone other than who they are. Your baby's character is then shaped by their experience of life.

Like adults and children, some babies cope with stress well, even thriving on it, whereas others are more sensitive, become quickly overwhelmed, or may even give up. The nature of your baby's personality and how he/she reacts and adjusts to the challenges of life will become clearer to you as they grow and develop. Essentially, we are who we are and we are shaped by our experiences.

Your baby is an active participant in being born. His/her body goes through physiological changes once labour is initiated and is actively involved in the potential journey through the birth canal. This means that they are not just a lump to be pushed out by you. If labour progresses well and naturally, birth becomes a synchronised process between the two of you.

Babies have a mind and are able to process thought at an early stage in their embryological development. As soon as enough nerves have grown and connected with each other in their developing brain, the processing of information becomes possible and some form of thought occurs. It is most likely that this occurs within two to four weeks of conception.

Thought processes in a baby are pre-verbal. This means that because they do not have speech, they don't think in words as we do, but their brains still think and that is why they are able to communicate. They know what's going on. Because a baby has thought, he/she also has the potential for brain memory.

Babies can develop a learned response or habit very early on, even in the womb. This is called imprinting. The sensory nerve pathways that are used first become the ones that shape their view of life and how they react to it. So if a baby's first experience of life is that it is a struggle, he/she may get the unconscious message that life is a struggle and then that is what it becomes. This could be why some babies find it so hard to settle. The same may be true for abandonment, pain, pleasure and love. Babies have the potential for over-riding original, learned responses.

As well as having brain memory, babies, and us as adults, have 'tissue memory'. This means that our body tissues such as muscles, fasciae (sheets of connecting tissue), fluids and bone have the ability to remember what happens to them, particularly when they are exposed to unpleasant outside forces such as impact, compression, pressure and puncture. This memory is held locally in the affected tissues and cells. It remains throughout life and is possible to recall non-verbally. Your baby's body holds within it the memory of what it experienced during and after birth. Some therapies work by accessing and processing tissue memory.

LIFE BEFORE BIRTH

It is widely accepted that babies have awareness in the womb. Babies in the womb have been shown to respond to familiar voices, sounds and music from outside their mother's body. This means your baby is aware of what he/she experiences while in your womb and also senses what is going on for you and around you. This sensory awareness is known as prenatal influence.

Babies in the womb are also understood to retain memory of their experience, but they may not know that they remember. This is pre-verbal memory. Do you remember what it was like to be in your mother's womb? The answer is most likely no, but then, as adults, we do spend much of our life creating womb-like spaces within which to feel secure.

The experiences you have during pregnancy, both pleasant and unpleasant, are also chemically experienced by your baby. Your growing baby's body will respond to events in your life by changes occurring in your body and blood chemistry. If you are feeling loved your body will release the hormone oxytocin, the love hormone, which will pass through your placenta into your baby and then he/she too will feel love. If, however, you are under pressure then your body will release stress hormones, which also pass to your baby and he/she may in turn feel activated and stressed too. This activation passes as you relax again.

WHEN YOUR BABY WON'T STOP CRYING

YOU HAVE MET THEIR NEEDS YET YOUR BABY STILL WON'T STOP CRYING

Difficulties may start for you as a parent when you are doing all the right things for your baby, meeting his/her needs as they arise, comforting them, and yet, they still don't settle, and continue to cry. Their crying may become excessive, inconsolable, or they may scream, even hysterically. The screaming may go on for hours at a time, with temporary respite perhaps while they are feeding, before carrying on again. This may become the same pattern every day and every night. The days merge into weeks and sometimes months.

This situation can become unbearable for any parent. You may hardly sleep, get no time to eat properly or rest, feel constantly tired, exhausted, irritable, and angry; at the end of your tether. It may be the same for your partner. Your relationship suffers and you have no normality to your life. Some parents go beyond their ability to cope, yet still carry on caring; you have no alternative. This can be torturous. Before, you did not know that looking after a baby could be this difficult. You may blame yourself and doubt your ability as a parent; though you are doing all you can and all that you know. Your friends and family may offer and give support, but they may not have an answer either and they are not living your life 24 hours a day.

IS SOMETHING ELSE WRONG?
When it is like this, parents often instinctively know that something is not right for their baby, but they may not know what it is. It may be clear that your baby is behaving as if he/she is in pain, but you don't know why.

Your baby is crying excessively, inconsolably, or screaming because they have issues other than need. Often it is beyond your personal resources as a parent to understand and resolve this situation. You need help.

DOES YOUR BABY HAVE OTHER SYMPTOMS?
If your baby does cry excessively or scream, he/she may display other symptoms or behaviour patterns too, which can give a health professional more idea of what is troubling them. Does your baby have any of these additional symptoms or behaviours:

- they struggle to feed well or they are intense feeders?
- they arch their neck and spine and go rigid when they cry or scream?
- they scream when you lie them on their back?

- their knees come up to their chest when they cry?
- they have difficulty turning their neck?
- they scream but settle once they have passed wind?
- their abdomen is rigid or bloated?
- they regularly bring up food, or vomit?
- they cry severely as soon as they start to feed and this may continue afterwards?
- they are fidgety and difficult to cuddle?
- they are always alert and have difficulty letting go to sleep?
- they wake at the slightest noise?
- they scream during sleep as if having a nightmare?
- they always wake crying?
- they cry angrily?
- they get worked up to the point they could explode?
- they fail to make good eye contact?
- they appear withdrawn or over-quiet?
- they never seem happy?

Your baby may show some or all of the above symptoms. If they do, it is time to seek professional help. Most of these symptom patterns can be explained and often helped or resolved.

ASKING FOR HELP

If your baby continues to cry excessively, inconsolably, or to scream, the first health professionals you need to talk to are your midwife and health visitor. They may make recommendations, but if nothing changes it is time to consult your doctor.

Hopefully your doctor will listen to you, hear what you are saying and not just treat you as an over-anxious mother. If, after examining your baby, they are able to reach a diagnosis, they may advise a course of action, or if they are still concerned, refer you to a paediatrician or hospital. However, in many cases mothers are told that their baby is fine, that they just have a crying baby, or that it is 'colic', and he/she will eventually grow out of it. If you get told this, it is of no immediate help.

If none of the medical advice, interventions or prescribed medications makes any difference, you may feel completely on your own. You have a crying and screaming baby, nobody knows why and nothing helps. But you are not alone: many parents find themselves in the same situation. It is helpful to ask around to see if other parents have similar issues with their baby and ask how they cope and whether they have come across anything else that helps.

YOUR BABY'S CRY FOR HELP

The first step is to acknowledge that your baby is crying excessively or screaming for a reason. Crying and screaming are communications that something is not right. The next step is to begin to learn more about what makes babies cry excessively, or scream. Usually there is an explanation for their behaviour and further help available. It is also important for you to look after yourself as best you can and to be looked after. You will need some time for rest and recuperation and may need to seek help and support from a partner, friends, family and health professionals. Do not be afraid to ask, particularly if you are struggling and feel alone.

Chapter 2.
WHY SOME BABIES CRY EXCESSIVELY OR SCREAM

This chapter reviews the main reasons why your baby might cry excessively or scream. If the reasons for your baby's upset are understood, it is easier to find the most appropriate way to help him/her. The main reasons why some babies cry excessively or scream are: they are still getting over the experience of their birth, they are in pain, they are ill, or they have a sensory processing issue. With some of these situations the upset is temporary only, so will not be the cause of an ongoing problem.

THEY ARE STILL EXPERIENCING THE EFFECTS OF THEIR BIRTH

THE MOST COMMON AND LARGELY UNRECOGNISED CAUSE OF EXCESSIVE CRYING AND SCREAMING IN BABIES.

The most common and largely unrecognised cause of excessive crying and screaming in babies is that they are still experiencing the effects of their birth. For some unknown reason it is generally assumed that once a baby is born, he/she is OK. If they appear normal, are breathing well, feeding and have a good APGAR score (the first test given to a newborn immediately after birth - Appearence, Pulse, Grimace, Activity, Respiration. Scored out of ten, seven and above is normal), they are passed as fit. In some cases this is far from the truth. They may be healthy, but this does not mean they are OK and it certainly does not mean that they have fully recovered from the effects of their birth.

A similar situation exists with victims of car accidents. In most car accidents, even high-speed impacts, no bones are broken. Afterwards, the driver can get out, walk around, may feel a bit shaken and have a slightly sore neck, but feel OK enough, decide they got away with it and carry on with life as if nothing has happened. This is actually denial and is part of the trauma response.

A year later, the victim may be off work with severe neck stiffness, headaches, low back pain, tiredness, anxiety and depression. The soft-tissue injuries sustained to the head, spine and nervous system in those few seconds of impact are severe and can have far-reaching and long-term consequences, especially if not recognised and treated adequately.

And so it is with babies. Of course everyone wants their baby to be OK, no matter what he/she has been through. What happened, how long it took, how intense it was, if there was foetal distress or intervention, separation … all these events can blur into insignificance once your baby is safely in your arms. Did anyone assess your baby for the impact the birth process had on him/her? What help did he/she receive to promote recovery and resolution?

WHAT HAPPENS
The reality is that many babies are still experiencing the strain, stress or trauma of their birth and it is because of this that they cry excessively or scream. Often there is a connection between what your baby experienced during and after birth and how unsettled he/she is now.

Every baby is unique, as is every birth. The following is an example of what a baby may experience.

YOUR BABY'S CRY FOR HELP

Imagine being a baby. You are lying comfortably in your mother's womb, warm, content and secure. The due date has passed, so birth is induced. Suddenly, the soft uterine walls around you contract more intensely and repetitively. Your soft body is squeezed from all sides, moving you downwards. Some contractions are so powerful that they cause pain. Gradually you lose sense of what's going on. After enduring hours of this you become stressed and your body releases adrenaline, triggering the fight or flight stress response, but you're not going anywhere soon. A state of panic and fear ensues; you feel out of control. When and how will this end?

Your head moulds and you move through a hole smaller than the size of your head. Your neck twists and you experience more pain as your head pushes past your mother's pelvis. Forceps take hold of the sides of your head. The pain is intense and you want to yell, but you are not breathing yet. With the final tug, you burst into the delivery room. The light is so intense that your eyes are blinded. Your life-giving cord is abruptly cut and you feel a sense of suffocation. Instinctively you grab your first breath and scream.

Caesarean section may be no easy option either, especially if it is used in an emergency.

SYMPTOMS BIRTH MAY CAUSE
The following is a list of symptoms and behaviours that many babies have that can be the effect of them not having completely recovered from the strain, stress, or trauma experienced during their birth process.

- **Excessive crying.** Excessive, severe, constant, or inconsolable crying. Cries for no apparent reason, or when put down.
- **Screaming.** Often hysterically. May be high-pitched as if in pain. Can go on for hours, sometimes all waking moments.
- **Trapped wind.** Difficult to wind after feeds, difficulty burping and farting. Trapped wind causes pain and screaming.
- **Digestive disturbances.** Colic, constipation, vomiting, reflux.
- **Excessive comfort feeding.** Wants to feed constantly, only content when feeding.
- **Feeding difficulties.** Struggles to feed well. Unable to synchronise feeding with breathing and swallowing.
- **Breathing issues.** Irregular, erratic, noisy or fast breathing; tight chest; baby asthma; cannot breathe well while sucking.

YOUR BABY'S CRY FOR HELP

- **Sleep disturbances.** Poor sleep day and/or night, fights going to sleep, easily disturbed, no long sleep. Wakes in the night screaming, cries on waking.
- **Clingyness.** Constant need to be held. Cries when put down, or if you leave the room.
- **Fractious and unsettled.** Always on edge and needing attention, rarely at peace.
- **Body spasms.** Arches spine, constantly pulls head backwards or brings knees up to chest.
- **Stiff neck.** Difficulty turning the neck one or both ways.
- **Rigid body.** Does not soften when held.
- **Exaggerated reflexes.** Very jumpy, startles easily.
- **Over-alert baby.** Always alert, fights sleep, won't let go, intense feeder, over-active and has constant need for stimulation.
- **Poor social engagement.** Poor eye contact, turns head away, disinterested; does not cry to be picked up.
- **Unhappy.** Rarely content, rarely smiles, grumpy. Looks and behaves as if unhappy or sad.
- **Being unresponsive.** Poor and disinterested feeder, sucks poorly, low body tone, unresponsive, rarely cries, excessive sleep.

You may be surprised and recognise some of these

patterns in your own baby. Many people consider the above as being normal for a baby and this is the point: these symptom patterns are normal for most babies because most babies are still suffering the stress, strain, or trauma of their birth. In practice, craniosacral therapists find that over 90% of babies retain in their body some effect from birth.

BABY GRIEF

Many babies and children are suffering from grief due to their birth. Grief is not something we experience only after bereavement; we also experience it when we have not got over something serious that happened. Grieving is a process of recovering from the shock, learning to accept what happened, processing it and then moving on. If we fail to get over something that happened, the grieving process is incomplete and the grief becomes held within us.

If your baby has not completely recovered from his/her birth process, he/she may have a pattern of held grief. A baby suffering from held grief may cry easily and excessively and be triggered into crying by insignificant events. They may cry inconsolably, as if their world has come to an end.

In an older baby or child held grief may show up as anxiety, lack of confidence, being easily upset, swallowing issues and breathing disorders, including asthma. Held grief tends to locate in the chest and diaphragm because it is essentially held-back tears – the mourning that never happened. This is the same for adults. Often, the first thing to release when treating a baby is their held grief, sometimes as tears.

A major difference between an adult experiencing something difficult and a baby during his/her birth is that the adult can vocalise. An adult is able to shout, scream, swear, or cry for help; a baby cannot. During birth, because the baby is getting its oxygen supply from its placenta and not by breathing, he/she is unable to use their voice. So when a baby in the womb, or birth canal, gets stressed, distressed, or is in pain, he/she cannot shout, cry, or scream. Instead their distressed emotions become held in their body.

THEY ARE IN PAIN

The other main reason why babies cry excessively or scream is because they are in pain. Inside and outside the womb, babies can feel pain because they have a brain, nerves and pain sensors (nociceptors). If your baby is in pain he/she will cry with a 'painful cry'. This is a severe, piercing cry or scream. Impossible to ignore, it can be distressing to listen to. Pain may come in bouts, or be continuous, in which case your baby may scream inconsolably for hours. This is a dreadful scenario for any parent to endure.

There are many reasons why a baby may experience pain; the following is an overview.

INJURY
Some babies experience injuries during birth that cause them to scream with pain afterwards. This is commonly due to head, neck and shoulder strains. Rarely, a baby sustains a fracture during birth, most often of a clavicle (collar bone), or skull bone. A baby with a painful physical injury is likely to scream more when moved. The screaming will ease as their body heals.

Physical injuries and fractures can also be sustained by a baby any time after birth, either accidentally, or intentionally. If your baby has sustained a physical injury that concerns you, you need to get them checked out by a doctor, or go to A&E.

Medical procedures may cause a baby pain and, if performed repetitively, can trigger their stress response. Taking blood samples, inserting a canula and feeding tubes, and performing a lumbar puncture cause pain – sometimes severe pain. This is why babies scream when undergoing these procedures. A medical procedure may be a baby's first ever experience of pain. Medical personnel now largely recognise that babies are capable of experiencing pain, even in the womb.

HEADACHES

The reality is that some babies experience a headache or head pain after birth, which may be ongoing. If your head had been compressed for hours and then squeezed through a tight hole, or clamped and pulled out with an instrument, it would be surprising if it did not hurt afterwards. It is difficult to tell if a baby has a headache. If your baby does not like his/her head being touched, or constantly bangs his/her head, this could be an indication of a headache or head pain.

__Case study 1__: A five-year-old boy presenting with behavioural problems. After his first treatment of cranial osteopathy he reported that his headache had gone, yet he had never complained of headaches. He never realised he had a headache before because it had always been there and so he had accepted this was normal. His behaviour improved too!

In many adults with a life-time history of headaches, the cause can often be traced back to a birth injury involving compression and twisting of the upper neck bones on the base of the skull, which is still present but can be treated.

WHY SOME BABIES CRY EXCESSIVELY

DIGESTIVE ISSUES
A digestive problem is a common cause of painful crying and screaming in babies. They may become inconsolable. This may occur as frequent and daily episodes. Trapped wind is the most frequent cause. If your baby has trapped wind they may have difficulty burping and farting; also trouble winding after a feed. When they burp or pass wind, they become more settled.

Other signs a baby is troubled by his/her digestion include: a tight or bloated abdomen, lots of gurgling noises, diarrhoea or constipation, vomiting and reflux. They may clench their hands, bring their knees up, or straighten out rigidly. If your baby has any of these symptoms, you may assume, or be told, that he/she has colic. But what is colic?

If you research a definition of colic, you will find something like this:

'Episodes of crying for more than three hours per day and more than three days per week in an otherwise healthy baby between the ages of two weeks and four months, for which there is no known cause'.

So when a baby is diagnosed with colic basically this means they are crying excessively, or screaming, but no one knows why.

Some babies diagnosed with colic do not have colic and do not actually have a digestive problem at all; they have been misdiagnosed. Their symptoms are due to other stress, strain and trauma effects of their birth, which they are still experiencing.

However, when babies do have genuine digestive symptoms of trapped wind, constipation, intestinal cramps, vomiting and minor reflux, the cause can still be traced to their birth because the birth process can upset the functioning of the digestive system. It does this in five main ways:

i. The stress of birth causing the baby to feed erratically, swallowing air.
ii. The stress of birth stimulating overactivity of the entire digestive system from the mouth to the anus as part of the fight or flight stress response.
iii. Strains to the base of the skull during delivery, upsetting the main nerve, which regulates the function of the digestive system; the vagus nerve.
iv. A baby's diaphragm holding tension after a stressful birth, upsetting the stomach.
v. Tension around the umbilicus from cutting the cord too early.

If your baby has digestive issues, he/she needs to be assessed to see if any of the above tension patterns are active in their body.

Extreme digestive issues may have a more medical basis, though – for example, severe gastro-oesophageal reflux disease (GORD). This is a dire condition, in which the valve between the stomach and oesophagus (food pipe) is not working properly and allows stomach acid to come up. The stomach acid enters the oesophagus, burning it and causing severe pain. Babies with this condition may scream intensely as soon as they start feeding, or afterwards. If your baby suffers like this, you will need to be referred to a paediatrician.

Some babies have problems with the valve between the stomach and the intestines (pyloric stenosis) preventing the stomach contents from emptying. This causes stomach swelling and vomiting. Usually it is diagnosed early on by a paediatrician because it interferes with normal feeding.

Blocking of the intestine can occur in babies (intussusception and volvulus). These are medical emergencies. A blockage will cause a sudden change in your baby, with severe screaming and vomiting. You may realise something is unusual and very wrong.

If you think your baby has serious digestive issues, you need to consult your doctor, who may refer you to a paediatrician. However, the majority of digestive issues in babies are due to disturbances in normal regulation linked to effects from birth. Often they can be helped. Immaturity of the digestive system could also be a factor in some babies, as can milk issues.

MILK ISSUES

Some form of milk intolerance is not unusual in babies. Milk intolerance may cause indigestion, bloating, excessive wind and painful crying. It is important to differentiate between two types of milk issue:

i. allergy to cow's milk
ii. lactose intolerance

Allergy to cow's milk is common and often runs in families. If your baby is allergic to cow's milk and you are not breastfeeding, your child may tolerate goat's milk or soya formula. If you are breastfeeding you may need to stop eating all milk products, because the milk proteins can come through your breast milk.

Lactose, also called 'milk sugar', is present in breast milk and cow's milk. The intestines of some babies lack the enzyme lactase, which breaks down the milk sugar during digestion. The lactose then ferments in the gut, causing bloating and pain. The solution is to give a baby lactase drops if they are breastfed, or to use a formula with added lactase.

TEETHING
Teething is a major reason for excessive crying and screaming in babies and can cause them, and you, much grief. As the teeth buds begin to grow within the confines of the hard gums they exert pressure, causing pain and so your baby cries. This may go on for months, even before the first tooth appears. As well as screaming intermittently, your teething baby may dribble constantly, have a red cheek or ear and want to chew on hard objects.

There is no wonder solution for teething; it is a case of experimenting with different remedies such as teething granules and teething gels. Your baby will get through this stage. Babies who are hypersensitive and those that became stressed during birth are less likely to cope well with teething pain, because their tolerance to pain is diminished.

ILLNESS

Babies become ill from time to time. An ill baby is likely to be fractious and to cry more than usual, though he/she may also sleep more. Acute illnesses are sudden in onset, temporary and unlikely to be the cause of ongoing or excessive crying, or screaming. Once your baby is better, his/her disposition should return to normal. However, it is important to know when to suspect a serious acute illness such as meningitis.

MENINGITIS

Meningitis is a concern as a possible cause of excessive crying and screaming in your baby if there is a sudden deterioration in his/her disposition and behaviour. You may quickly realise that something is very wrong. If you find yourself in this situation, do not doubt your natural instincts and seek medical help immediately.

A baby with meningitis may have any or all of the following signs and symptoms but not necessarily all at the same time:

- fever, possibly with cold hands and feet
- no appetite, refusing food, or even vomiting
- dislike of being handled, fretfulness
- a high-pitched moaning sound, or whimpering
- they bend their neck backwards with arching of the spine
- a blank, staring expression
- lethargy, listless; difficult to wake
- pale, blotchy complexion

- a rash, spots or bruises that do not turn white when pressed

If you think your baby is displaying of the above symptoms, telephone your doctor immediately, or take him/her to hospital, because meningitis develops rapidly and can be life threatening. Should the symptoms be dismissed as a common cold but your instinct tells you otherwise, get an immediate second opinion. Time is of the essence with meningitis.

OTHER ACUTE ILLNESS
Your baby is naturally open to acute illness and infections as his/her immune system is still developing in response to life outside the womb. In most instances these are naturally self-limiting and do not require treatment, though it is essential to keep your baby's fluid intake up when ill because he/she can quickly become dehydrated.

There are various acute illnesses that affect babies such as coughs, colds, measles, mumps, rubella and chicken pox. Some babies are prone to recurrent high temperatures, which quickly subside with no cause being found. Earache is uncommon in a young baby.

When your baby is acutely ill, he/she may lose their appetite, develop a high temperature, be unusually fretful and cry, or scream more than usual; they could also be unusually quiet and sleep more. If an acute illness is causing symptoms that concern you, or is not clearing up, you need to consult your doctor. However, an acute illness is not going to be the cause of ongoing excessive crying and screaming. Your doctor's surgery should have further information about acute childhood illnesses including meningitis available for you.

Some babies develop an acute illness a few days after a vaccination. Typically this involves a high temperature, an increase in fretfulness, disturbed sleep patterns and upset digestion. Usually this settles on its own. If you consult your doctor when you suspect your baby has a vaccination reaction, most likely you will be told he/she has caught a cold and that it is a coincidence.

SERIOUS MEDICAL ILLNESS

If your baby has a serious illness this will usually have been picked up by your health visitor, doctor or paediatrician. A serious illness will have additional symptoms, such as lethargy, tiredness, pallor, poor appetite and failure to thrive. Excessive crying and screaming may not be part of this.

GENETIC DISORDERS

Genetic disorders are rare. They may not be diagnosed in a newborn unless the baby's physical appearance indicates a possible genetic anomaly. A genetic disorder may be considered as a diagnosis by a paediatrician at a later stage once it is clear that the infant's growth, development and behaviour is following an unusual and inexplicable pattern. A child later diagnosed with a genetic disorder could have been a more difficult baby.

SENSORY PROCESSING ISSUES

Our brains constantly receive and filter all the sensory information that comes from the sense organs of our bodies. The brain then reacts to this information accordingly and hopefully appropriately. Our main sense organs are our special senses of sight, smell, taste, hearing and touch. We also have special sense organs, which are microscopic nerve endings (proprioceptors) all over our body. These sensors constantly monitor pain, pressure, temperature, limb position and posture and send this information to the brain. This process is known as proprioception. All of this occurs automatically; we do not have to think about it. The main processing part of our brain is the 'mid-brain', particularly a structure called the thalamus.

SENSORY PROCESSING DISORDERS
A sensory processing disorder occurs when:

- too much sensory information is arriving at the brain and it is failing to cope
- the brain's sensory filters are not working well enough, so too much information gets through
- the brain is slow in processing, or fails to process even the normal amount of arriving sensory information
- there is a history of trauma

Either way the result is overwhelm. If you were to perceive all the sensory information that arrives at your brain each second, it would blow your mind! Unfortunately, this is what life is like for some people, including some children and babies. This is why the brain has filters to modify the excessive amount of sensory input, to make life tolerable and a pleasure.

If a baby, especially a very young baby, has a sensory processing issue he/she can become overwhelmed by the slightest thing. This includes being over-handled, busy and noisy environments, bright lights; sometimes even the mouth sensation of feeding can be too much. When a baby becomes overwhelmed he/she is likely to cry excessively and inconsolably because they are failing to cope.

Some people are born with a sensory processing disorder. This develops during the growth of their brain in the womb and remains so throughout their life.

Sensory processing disorders can result from head or brain injury, where parts of the brain are damaged and lose their ability to function normally. They can also be the result of mental or emotional trauma, including attachment disorders with babies, where the victim is left over-sensitised. A mechanical strain to the base of the skull can interfere with the easy nerve communication between the two sides of the brain and slow brain processing, resulting in sensory overload. This type of strain commonly occurs during birth and can be resolved by treating the strain using craniosacral therapy or cranial osteopathy.

BRAIN IMMATURITY

A baby's immature brain is still developing. New nerves are constantly being formed and are growing and making connections with other nerves. Because of this a baby's brain has a limit to how much sensory information it can process. If the birth process is very intense, or very long, the baby's brain may become overloaded by the pressure and pain information it receives and then go into overwhelm. What a baby feels in this situation is that it is all too much and he/she wants it to stop. If a baby is in overwhelm and labour is still progressing, or he/she is stuck, they may tip into becoming traumatised. If a baby in such a situation also has a developmental sensory processing disorder, he/she will get overwhelmed at a much earlier stage.

Newborns still stressed by the effects of their birth process may also become overwhelmed once they are born because they find the sensory input from their environment, such as light, noise and hustle, too much to cope with. This sensory overload particularly applies to very premature babies because they have little protection from the harsh sensory reality of the world outside the womb. Overwhelmed babies can be helped.

NATURAL HYPERSENSITIVITY
Some people are naturally hypersensitive. If you are hypersensitive as an adult, most likely you were as a baby and child too. It may initially be tricky to spot if your baby is hypersensitive. If either you or their father is hypersensitive, they may be too. Hypersensitive babies very quickly go into meltdown, even if something is not drastically wrong. For example, when they become hungry they scream straight away, or they will go ballistic when you put them down or give them to someone else to hold. Usually they soon calm down once safely back with you.

A hypersensitive baby is usually happy most of the time; they just have episodes of severe screaming, but usually are not in pain. The hypersensitivity is not something they can help and needs to be respected. A hypersensitive baby is not a good candidate to try controlled crying with. (Controlled crying is a type of sleep training where babies are soothed and then left to cry for gradually lengthening periods of time. It is not recommended for babies under six months old).

AUTISTIC SPECTRUM DISORDERS (ASD)
It is generally understood that autistic spectrum disorders, such as autism and Asperger's Syndrome begin in the womb as the baby's brain is developing and as such they become part of that individual's nature. There is evidence to suggest that autism can also be triggered by factors after birth too, but mainly with susceptible babies and children.

It is highly unlikely that a health professional is going to consider a diagnosis of ASD in a baby who cries excessively or screams because there will not be enough clinical evidence to confirm this. These conditions become apparent as the infant grows and develops. Then, certain behavioural traits become more obvious. However, a later diagnosis of ASD in a child does often explain why they cried and screamed so much as a baby. As a newborn they may have been totally overwhelmed by life because of their hypersensitivity and sensory processing issues.

Some babies who cry and scream excessively also show a behavioural pattern of not making good eye contact, turning away, being unaffectionate and generally being difficult to engage with. This is most likely to be a social engagement issue and not an ASD, though it may initially be difficult to distinguish between the two because the presentations are similar. The most common reason for poor social engagement in a baby is trauma at, or after, birth. This could be caused by foetal distress, intervention, poor ventilation, separation, medical procedures, baby surgery, prematurity, incubation, adoption or neglect.

Chapter 3

HOW THE EFFECTS OF BIRTH CAN CAUSE YOUR BABY TO CRY

Most of the symptoms that occur in unsettled babies and those who cry excessively or scream can be explained by understanding how their body became upset during the birth process. This chapter looks at some useful physiology and then at understanding how the strain, stress and trauma issues that may arise during birth may still be affecting your baby now.

SOME USEFUL PHYSIOLOGY

Having knowledge of how your body works is helpful in

understanding your health, the health of your baby and why symptoms arise.

BONES AND JOINTS
The bones of our skull are called cranial bones and there are 21 of them. The bigger, plate-like bones make up the top, back, sides and floor of our skull. There is a complex of smaller bones that form our face, eye sockets, palate and upper jaw.

Joints are formed where the cranial bones meet each other. These joints are called sutures and remain throughout life – your head never fuses into one solid bone.

Joints exist in our body to allow movement. Movement in joints such as our knees, elbows and fingers is obvious, because we can watch them bend. Movement in the joints between our cranial bones is not obvious because we cannot see or feel them move, but they do move. This movement allows our skull to expand and contract subtly to allow for the movement of our brain and for fluid pressure changes within our skull. It can be felt by trained hands.

EFFECTS OF BIRTH CAN CAUSE YOUR BABY TO CRY

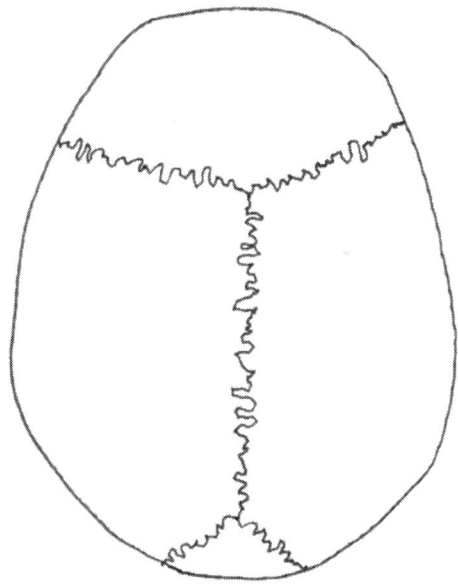

Figure 1. The cranial sutures. These joints between the cranial bones have an irregular shape. They allow movement and remain throughout life.

In babies, the joints between the main skull bones are not yet properly formed. This allows them to slide over each other during labour, so reducing the diameter of the head and making it easier to pass through their mother's pelvis during birth. This is the process of moulding.

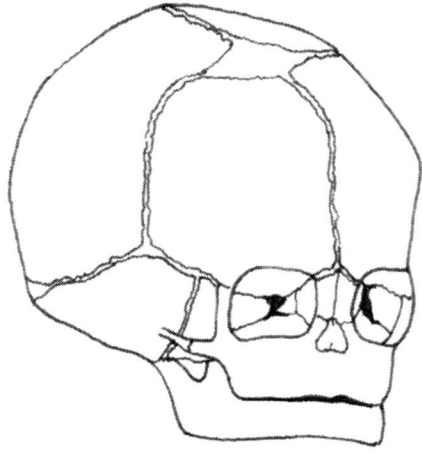

Figure 2. A newborn baby's skull. The sutures are not yet fully formed. This creates the 'soft spots', the fontanelles.

Because our cranial bones move slightly in relation to each other, they also have the potential to twist and become stuck. This gives some insight into what may happen to a baby's head during birth. If two or more bones become jammed together, they may not release completely afterwards, interfering with how well the brain and nervous system perform.

The sacrum is the bone that forms the back of our pelvic girdle, on top of which sits our spine. The sacrum and pelvis have a special relationship with the cranial bones. They are linked by the structure of the spine and move together in a synchronised pattern.

BRAINS, MEMBRANES AND FLUID
Our central nervous system is the control centre of our body and can be considered as five parts:

i. Our spinal cord, enclosed within our spine.
ii. Our brain stem, which is the thickening of the top of our spinal cord as it meets our brain. This is the most primitive part of our brain and is involved with our survival and stress responses. It is an active part of a baby's brain and is where our early reflexes come from.
iii. Our mid-brain, above the brain stem, which is the sensory processing centre and includes the thalamus.
iv. Our two brain hemispheres, right and left, which are our thinking and control centres. These two hemispheres are curled-up hollow tubes filled with fluid.

Lining our skull bones and surrounding our brain and spinal cord is a tough, sheet-like membrane called the dural membrane. This membrane helps to protect the brain and stabilises its movement within the skull. The dural membrane absorbs the compressive forces from labour and birth and can become tense and twisted, pressurising the brain.

The dural membrane is one of three membrane layers surrounding the brain, which make up the meninges. It is the meninges that become inflamed in meningitis.

The middle part of our brain and spinal cord are filled with a special fluid called the cerebrospinal fluid (CSF). This fluid also surrounds the outside of our brain and our spinal cord. The CSF is separated from our blood by the blood-brain barrier. This prevents infections in our blood stream reaching our brain. It is CSF that is drawn off when someone has a lumbar puncture.

The CSF protects, supports and provides nutrition for our brain. Put simply, our brain floats in this fluid. The CSF moves in two ways: it circulates within and around the brain and spinal cord and it moves in a tide-like pattern, ebbing and flowing like the sea. This movement pattern is known as cranial-sacral motion. It can be felt by trained hands and observed during brain and spinal surgery. Birth can upset the circulation and tidal motion of the CSF.

THE AUTONOMIC NERVOUS SYSTEM (ANS)
In addition to thinking, our brain operates our body using two main systems:

i. The somatic nervous system, which controls our muscles, movement and posture and is under our conscious control.
ii. The autonomic nervous system, which regulates how the insides of our body work; our organs, our special senses and the movement of blood. It is not under conscious control; it works automatically.

Knowing about our autonomic nervous system (ANS) helps us to understand some of the symptoms babies show.

The ANS also operates using two systems, these are:

i. **the parasympathetic nervous system,** which controls our resting state and digestion
ii. **the sympathetic nervous system,** which controls our fight or flight stress response

When we are resting, our parasympathetic nervous system is operating. This causes our heart and lungs to actively slow down, withdraws blood from our muscles, promotes recovery and repair and regulates the activity in our digestive system. Hence, we digest food better when we are relaxed.

If we get threatened or stressed then our sympathetic nervous system takes over. Combined with the release of adrenaline, our heart rate increases, breathing deepens, our muscles pump up with blood (for running), tissue repair and digestion is suspended (so we may urinate, defecate, or vomit), our brain goes on alert, pupils narrow and our hearing becomes more acute. We are now in fight or flight mode. Hence, when babies become distressed during birth, their heart speeds up and they may release meconium (the first poo).

CRANIAL NERVES
Many pairs of nerves come from our spinal cord and travel into our arms and legs. These are called spinal nerves. An example is the sciatic nerve which passes from our lower back and sacrum down the back of our legs. Spinal disc pressure on a sciatic nerve causes sciatica.

There is another group of nerves called cranial nerves. Cranial nerves are a collection of 12 pairs of nerves and they originate from our brain stem. They supply our organs of special sense and so are involved with sight, hearing, taste and smell. They also control the movements of our eyes, tongue, throat and some neck muscles and some of the functioning of our autonomic nervous system.

One particular cranial nerve, called the vagus nerve, travels from the base of our skull into our body and regulates most of our organs, including our heart, lungs, stomach and intestines. The normal functioning of the vagus nerve is crucial in babies.

In order to get to where they are going, cranial nerves must pass through little holes in the cranial bones called foramina. This is important because some of these foramina are situated at the suture between two cranial bones, so if the bones twist, or become jammed, the nerve may be affected.

There is a link between the cranial nerves and some of the symptoms of babies. For example, if the function of the cranial nerves is upset during birth, this may interfere with normal breathing, sucking, swallowing and digestion.

MECHANICAL STRAIN ISSUES ARISING DURING THE BIRTH PROCESS

Most injuries that our bodies sustain involve an impact, compression, twisting, or a combination of these forces. If intense enough, these strains will be absorbed into our body structure as tissue memory, creating patterns of tightness and contraction.

A natural birth is very much about repetitive compressing, moulding and twisting forces and occasionally impact. Marked mechanical strains in babies can cause symptoms including excessive crying or screaming due to pain, tension or cranial nerve disturbances.

COMPRESSION STRAINS
The nature of labour is compression. If your baby had a natural birth, his/her head and body will have been subjected to compression with each uterine contraction, the force increasing as labour progresses. This leads to moulding. Further compression may occur as he/she descends through your birth canal during delivery.

Compression of the skull during labour and birth is resisted by the cerebrospinal fluid, a hydraulic effect. Despite this, compression strains are often absorbed into the baby's cranial bones, dural membrane and even his/her brain. Once birth is over, the baby's body and head will naturally expand, but sometimes this process is incomplete and some compression remains. Expansion is aided by sucking, and particularly by breastfeeding.

Compression strains occur when the forces of compression do not release naturally after birth. They are most common after a short or intense labour, a long labour, following induction or the use of forceps. Compression does not occur with an elective caesarean birth, but does with an emergency caesarean because the baby will have experienced some labour.

A compression strain is likely to unsettle a baby, causing him/her to be irritable and to affect their ability to let go, relax and sleep well. A compressed head may look and feel tight and could be painful to the baby. A baby whose head produces much heat may have a compression strain.

The bones of the base of the skull, called the occiput, the sphenoid and the two temporal bones (which house the middle and inner ear), are more solid than the other cranial bones and are unable to mould. Because of this, if the base of the skull gets compressed during birth, often it does not release well afterwards.

Severe compression of the base of the skull can cause marked behavioural issues in babies and children because of the proximity to the brain stem. Compression of the sides of the skull affects the temporal bones and can lead to hyperactivity, poor sleep and difficulty switching off in babies and ear problems in infants and children.

If the face is compressed during birth the sinuses, palate and jaw can all be affected. This could interfere with nasal breathing, sucking and feeding.

During birth a baby's body is also subjected to compression. Compression strains commonly involve the neck, shoulders, torso and pelvis, while compression of the ribcage and diaphragm may interfere with the baby's ability to breathe normally and complicates digestion causing vomiting, reflux and trapped wind.

TWISTING AND BACKWARD BENDING STRAINS
Your baby's head, neck and body go through a twisting and backward bending (extension) motion as they descend through the birth canal. Sometimes this strain pattern does not fully release after birth. Signs of a twisting and backward bending strain in a baby include:

- an out-of-shape head
- difficulty turning the neck one, or both ways
- arching of the neck
- repetitive arching of the spine
- a twisted body
- crying triggered by being placed on his/her back
- problems with sucking, breathing, swallowing and the digestive system

EFFECTS OF BIRTH CAN CAUSE YOUR BABY TO CRY

The most common and serious twisting strain in babies involves the joints forming the base of the skull (the cranial base) and between the base of the skull and the top of the neck (sub-occipital joint). Severe strain of these joints, especially if it also involves compression and backward bending, can really upset a baby.

Cranial base and sub-occipital strain may make a baby repetitively arch his/her neck and spine. This is a reflex they cannot help and may affect feeding. They may be in pain and cry excessively or scream. Because this is the area where the brain stem enters the brain, a strain here can upset the balance of the nervous system causing tension, fretfulness, unsettledness, alertness, fear, sleep disturbances and increased reflexes and could trigger the stress response. The cranial nerve (called the vagus nerve) descends through the sub-occipital area, so a mechanical strain here can interfere with its normal function. This can directly cause digestive, heart and breathing symptoms. Some osteopaths believe that 80% of colic-type symptoms are caused by cranial base and sub-occipital irritation of the vagus nerve.

YOUR BABY'S CRY FOR HELP

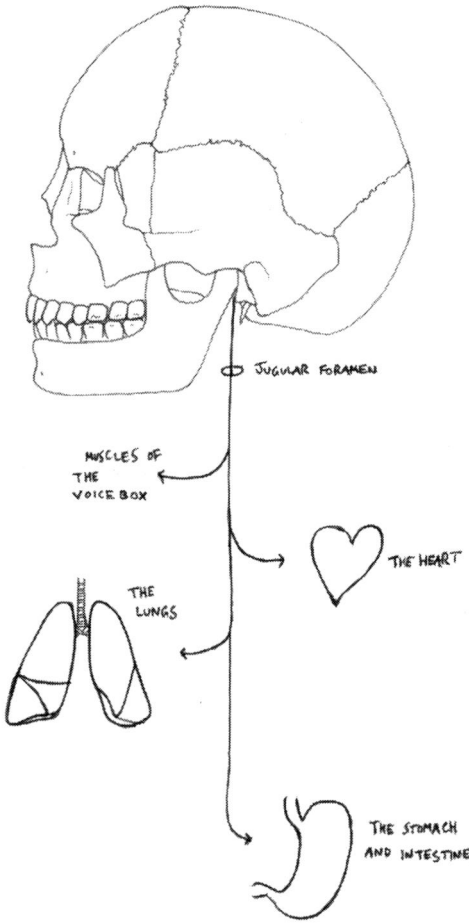

Figure 3. The vagus nerve. The vagus nerve descends through a foramina (opening) in the base of the skull, through the neck and into the torso. It supplies and regulates most of the body organs including our lungs, heart, stomach and intestines.

EFFECTS OF BIRTH CAN CAUSE YOUR BABY TO CRY

DURAL MEMBRANE STRAINS
Because the cranial bones of the top, back and sides of a newborn's head are not yet fully formed, resistance of the skull largely comes from the dural membranes. These membranes absorb much of the compression and twisting forces during labour and birth. If the skull is out of shape or compressed, the dural membranes are always involved as well as the bones.

Tight dural membranes in a baby can create tension in his/her brain, making it more reactive and affecting the ability to process information well, resulting in overload. A baby with compressed membranes may cry more, be more fretful, harder to please and may have angry outbursts. They are like a bear with a sore head!

CRANIAL NERVE INJURIES IN BABIES
Cranial nerve problems are common in babies and are often the cause of digestive disturbances, feeding and breathing problems.

Because the cranial nerves follow pathways through the foramina (holes) in cranial bones and between cranial bones, mechanical strains involving the cranial bones and their dural membrane lining may adversely affect how these nerves are firing. This is particularly relevant in the base of the skull, upper neck and face – areas frequently compressed during birth.

The most important cranial nerves for babies are those involved with the mouth, face, throat, neck, special senses and the functioning of the heart, lungs and digestive system. These include:

- the trigeminal nerve, which controls the muscles of sucking and of the throat
- the facial nerve, which controls facial expression and the production of tears
- the auditory nerve, which modifies hearing
- the hypoglossal nerve, which raises the throat in speaking and swallowing
- the vagus nerve, which supplies the heart, lungs and organs of the digestive system
- the accessory nerve, which moves the throat, soft palate, neck and shoulders
- the glossopharyngeal nerve, which controls the movement of the tongue in sucking, swallowing and speaking

Of particular note is that the vagus, hypoglossal and accessory nerves all go through the same foramen in the base of the skull, called the jugular foramen. So a compression or twisting strain of the base of the skull could narrow this foramen and upset all these nerves together. This does happen. Cranial nerves are also involved with the functioning of the autonomic nervous system.

EFFECTS OF BIRTH CAN CAUSE YOUR BABY TO CRY

If your baby struggles to suck, feed, or swallow well, has a problem co-ordinating feeding, breathing and swallowing, makes few facial expressions, turns away, or has breathing or digestive symptoms, this could be due to interference with his/her cranial nerves and is frequently caused by birth strains.

Cranial nerve issues often resolve once any mechanical or compressive strains around the base of the skull, face, and upper neck have been treated and resolved.

Mechanical strains are responsible for many unsettled behaviours in babies and if severe, could cause excessive crying. Because of the close relationship between the skull, brain, neck and spinal cord, mechanical strains here can affect the activity level of the spinal cord, triggering alertness and increased reflex activity.

Understanding the relationship between the skull and the cranial nerves also explains many of the symptoms young babies have. It takes a specialised therapist to be able to evaluate and treat a baby for compression and strain issues. Doctors do not usually do this. These therapists are called craniosacral therapists and cranial osteopaths.

THE STRESSED BABY

Understanding how we respond to and are affected by stress is essential for understanding babies, because many of the symptoms that arise in newborns are caused by an active stress response. Some babies cry excessively or scream because they are still stressed from their birth experience.

THE STRESS RESPONSE
Life is a series of constant challenges. Some challenges we choose, others come out of the blue. Prepared or not, we need to be able to respond to them all.

The human body is equipped with a system that helps it respond healthily to challenging events. This system is called the stress response and falls under the control of the sympathetic nervous system. The stress response evolved over millions of years to enable creatures to cope with life- threatening situations. Many of the stresses we face today are not life-threatening, but this same system is triggered.

The stress response prepares us for potential danger, for fight or flight. When the danger has passed, and we are safe again, the stress response should settle and we return to the resting state. Problems arise when a challenging situation becomes too much and the stress response continues, even after the stressful challenge has passed. Then the body is left in a state of heightened alertness and readiness; we say we are stressed.

Challenging situations occur when we feel unsafe, when we have too little space, when we are threatened, when events go on for too long, or are too intense. This also describes what many babies experience during birth.

BABIES AND STRESS
The stress response may be triggered in your baby. This may occur if his/her birth process becomes painful, too intense, goes on for too long, he/she becomes stuck, or when interventions are used. An induced birth is more stressful to a baby due to its suddenness and intensity.

During birth babies also respond to their mother's experiences and to their environment. If their mother becomes stressed by going into hospital or during the birth process, or if the hospital environment is fraught, the baby will sense this too.

When mothers become stressed during birth, labour slows down and may even stop. This is because the fight or flight stress response causes labour to cease. The stress response, however, speeds up delivery. This explains why labour often stops when a mother arrives in hospital and how she is suddenly able to push her baby out when the obstetrician goes off to get the forceps.

When a baby becomes stressed during birth, his/her sympathetic nervous system triggers the stress response. Then the heart rate increases, blood rushes to his/her muscles and he/she becomes alert as the body prepares for fight or flight. Unfortunately for a baby, he/she is unable to fight or flee, so the stress tension builds up in their body and nervous system. It is this stress that may not release after birth, leaving the baby alert and tense.

If, however, both mother and baby are able to remain in the resting state during birth, the parasympathetic nervous system stays in control and labour progresses well and naturally. This is why births often progress better if the mother is at ease in a safe, warm, pleasant and familiar environment, such as home. However, hospitals and birthing pools can create the same feeling of relaxation and safety.

SIGNS OF STRESS IN A BABY
The signs that a baby is stressed are the same as for adults. If your child displays any of the following signs, he/she may be suffering from an active stress response:

EFFECTS OF BIRTH CAN CAUSE YOUR BABY TO CRY

- a tense body
- regular and excessive crying
- digestive issues
- fast or irregular heart rate
- irregular breathing
- a tight chest or asthma
- poor sleep, difficulty falling asleep, frequent waking
- unsettledness and fractiousness
- always on edge, or alert
- anxious or fearful
- have a need to be held constantly
- regular comfort feeding

With many babies the stress response naturally triggers during the challenge of being born and then calms down quickly afterwards. This process is helped by skin contact, feeding and a feeling of security.

It is the babies who become stressed and are unable to relax well after birth that remain tense and alert and may go on to develop symptoms of stress, including excessive crying. Additional mechanical strains may prevent the stress response from settling. It is therapeutically possible to help release the stress response in a baby so he/she calms down and settle into the resting state.

THE ANGRY BABY
Some babies are angry. Such babies may have no patience and quickly become frustrated. An angry baby will cry with an angry cry. They may even go ballistic, or totally out of control; the anger can become rage. When an angry baby calms, he/she too will wonder what has just happened. It is helpful to acknowledge if your baby is angry.

Anger is a natural expression of frustration and is often the response to being trapped in a difficult circumstance, particularly one from which you cannot escape. For an adult this could be putting up with a bad job or being stuck in a difficult relationship.

And so it is with babies. If the birth process becomes too intense, too long, too painful, the baby becomes stuck, or if forceps are used, he/she may become stressed and angry. If you were stuck with your head painfully squashed in a tight hole for many hours, even a day, you would become angry too!

Because babies in the womb and birth canal are not yet breathing, they are unable to express their anger by shouting and screaming, so it gets trapped inside their body as tissue memory. After birth this anger remains inside them; it does not just disappear. Once such babies are born and find their voice they will vent this anger at any opportunity; they may be unable to cry gently. An angry baby is a baby with anger held in his/her body but angry babies can be helped.

A caesarean baby may be angry too. If he/she was happy in the womb and was not ready to come out, they may be really upset by being pulled out without prior warning.

An angry baby may become an angry child and adult. Angry teenagers and adults may still have anger trapped inside their body from their birth.

Case study 2: *A 16-year-old presented with stress and anger issues, and a history of headaches. Assessment revealed severe head and upper neck compression (he has no internal space) and a chronic stress response. This strain and stress pattern is due to his birth. The client's mother confirmed his difficult delivery.*

After just one craniosacral therapy treatment, client reports being calmer, having a different attitude, no episodes at school and did not get angry for two weeks. Mother reports client being calmer too.

THE TRAUMATISED BABY

UNDERSTANDING TRAUMA

Trauma is the stage beyond stress. The physiological function of trauma is to separate the individual from an intolerable situation so he/she can survive it. An intolerable situation may not be life-threatening but is unbearable. Examples include abandonment, imprisonment, abuse and ongoing severe physical, emotional, or mental pain.

During trauma the body remains physically present to what is going on and may even be injured or damaged, but the individual has withdrawn mentally and emotionally because he/she can no longer cope. They become dissociated from their body, or retreat deep within, where they can no longer be hurt.

Trauma mode is a primitive function of the parasympathetic nervous system, the control of which arises from our brain stem. The brain stem is often called the reptilian brain because it was the first part of the brain to evolve, and controls the survival reflexes. Going into trauma is a survival reflex.

Reptiles and some animals, especially small, fluffy animals like rabbits, go into trauma when attacked by a predator. They are unable to fight or to run quickly away, so they

EFFECTS OF BIRTH CAN CAUSE YOUR BABY TO CRY

freeze, shut down, play dead. Because predators enjoy a fight, if their prey is unresponsive and appears to be dead, they lose interest and wander off. Several minutes later, once the coast is clear, the victim begins to come round. They shake, get up and then carry on as if nothing has happened.

This same process occurs in humans as a means of surviving extreme situations. However, unlike animals, humans, including babies, often do not come completely out of the freeze response, so remain shut down and detached. This is the state of 'post-trauma'.

The state of trauma may trigger in a baby when the birth process exceeds the normal range of events and the stress response fails to be enough to get them through. Ongoing stress, mechanical strain, compression, pain, or fear become intolerable due to their intensity, severity, or duration. For the baby the experience of his/her birth has become unbearable; they are totally over-whelmed, fail to cope and their primitive nervous system drops into the trauma mode. The unbearable nature of their situation may continue but at a deeper level the suffering is no longer felt; the baby survives.

Most babies do not go into trauma during birth. Those who do show particular symptoms and behaviours and will need professional help.

SIGNS OF TRAUMA IN A BABY AND THEIR FAMILY
Any or all of the following may be happening when a baby is suffering from trauma:

- severe and constant crying, or screaming, often hysterically. Likely to be a painful scream, though he/she may not be in physical pain. Can be inconsolable for hours. You will not be able to tell what is wrong
- easily becomes overwhelmed and goes into repetitive behaviours which they cannot switch off
- won't be put down without screaming, baby may need to be held constantly
- likely to express anger, or rage
- excessive and constant feeding or much comfort feeding. May only be quiet while feeding or may not be interested in feeding at all
- will often have severe colic-like symptoms and other digestive disturbances, including severe reflux, for which they may already be on medication
- may have been quiet or subdued for the first few weeks of life before becoming very upset
- appears distant or detached; avoids eye contact. Late to smile or rarely smiles. No facial expressions. May be undemonstrative as an infant
- severe sleep disturbances. Constantly alert,

EFFECTS OF BIRTH CAN CAUSE YOUR BABY TO CRY

hyper-vigilant and fights going to sleep. May sleep well at night, or hardly at all. Momentary naps during the day, if at all. May scream during sleep; suffers night terrors. Wakes screaming
- parents are driven to complete distraction, often feeling unable to cope
- parents often traumatised too and the mother may have a greater tendency towards developing postnatal depression
- recurrent visits to GP, or A&E, due to parental concerns, but nothing found to be wrong
- as an infant he/she may develop obsessive-type behaviour and demand a routine

If you recognise this pattern of extreme behaviour in your baby, it is likely that he/she is suffering from trauma. You may wish to discuss this with your doctor or paediatrician, though medical acknowledgement of trauma in babies is unusual. Many craniosacral therapists and cranial osteopaths are experienced at assessing and working with traumatised babies.

SITUATIONS THAT MAY CAUSE A BABY TRAUMA
The trauma response may be triggered in a baby during or after birth and includes the following situations:

- a very prolonged labour, especially if the baby has become stuck

- when the baby has experienced severe ongoing pain. This includes difficult forceps extraction
- when the baby experiences their birth as being totally out-of-control
- when the baby has failed to breathe, or stopped breathing altogether after delivery
- following repetitive painful medical procedures and as a complication of baby surgery
- in a medical emergency, such a foetal distress and emergency caesarean section, especially if forceps are used to extract the baby during the caesarean
- when the mother has become traumatised
- when a baby has been separated from his/her mother for too long after birth
- baby adoption
- prematurity: the majority of very premature babies suffer trauma. Going into the trauma mode is how they survive, especially if much time is spent in neonatal intensive care
- situations of abuse and neglect. A neglected infant may appear to be OK because he/she is quiet – in fact they have withdrawn

If your baby has experienced any of the above scenarios during or after birth, they may well show signs of trauma.

EFFECTS OF BIRTH CAN CAUSE YOUR BABY TO CRY

TRAUMA AND POOR SOCIAL ENGAGEMENT

Human beings are a highly evolved species. As such, we are social creatures – we live in social groups. In order to socialise, we have evolved a social engagement system. This is a neurologically based system that controls how we orientate to others (turn our head), our facial expressions, how we make eye contact, how we listen and our vocal expression. We are hard-wired to be social.

It is our parasympathetic nervous system that controls our social engagement system – the same system that triggers during trauma, hence the relationship between the two.

When a baby goes into trauma, his/her social engagement system may cut off too. This effect is mediated by the cranial nerves that control the neck, mouth, tongue and eye movement, facial expressions and hearing. The result is that the baby turns away, is expressionless, avoids eye contact and is unusually quiet. This is an automatic response, a reflex. A traumatised baby cannot help this behaviour and it is not to be confused with autism.

When a baby comes out of trauma, he/she will begin to turn their neck more (orientate), make better eye contact, become more facially expressive and more vocal. They may begin to tremble and to cry and scream for the first time – a healthy response in this situation.

YOUR BABY'S CRY FOR HELP

Caring for a baby suffering from trauma may be hard work; it can be difficult to cope with but he/she cannot help how they are. Their body and mind are under the control of their parasympathetic nervous system, a primitive survival response. You are helping your baby just by being with them. Creating a safe and consistent environment, skin-to-skin contact, talking gently, or singing and encouraging eye contact will help too. Traumatised babies can be helped therapeutically, but there is no quick fix.

Understanding some physiology and the mechanical strain, stress and trauma reactions that occur in babies during and after birth helps to explain many of their symptom patterns and behaviours, especially in those babies who cry excessively or scream.

Chapter 4
HOW YOUR BABY EMERGED INTO THE WORLD

Whatever a baby has experienced during his/her birth process, there is something profound about how they emerge into the world. We are all affected by our birth, whether we realise this or not. This chapter considers the different ways babies enter the world and the events of the postnatal period.

NATURAL DELIVERY

BIRTH AND THE AUTONOMIC NERVOUS SYSTEM
When the time arrives, the onset of labour is triggered by release of the hormone oxytocin, which comes from the mother's pituitary gland in the brain. It may be her body that triggers this release, or signals from the

baby's; most likely it is a combination of the two. Oxytocin causes the uterus to contract, initiating labour. It is also the hormone given in inductions, to artificially initiate the onset of labour.

The progress of labour is another function of the autonomic nervous system. Here, there is an evolutionary story to tell:

> *Cavewoman is relaxed and feels safe crouching behind a bush. Her labour is progressing fine (a parasympathetic nervous system response). Woolly mammoth appears. Cavewoman feels threatened and goes into fight or flight. Labour abruptly stops (a sympathetic nervous system response) and she runs off to find safety. Once safe, her body drops back into her resting state and labour continues (the parasympathetic nervous system response again).*

> *Cavewoman enters second stage. Delivery of cave baby is imminent. Suddenly, sabre-toothed tiger turns up. Cavewoman's body goes into fight or flight. Second stage is speeded up dramatically (a different sympathetic nervous system response), cave baby pops out; mother cradles him and runs off to find safety. Once safe again, the placenta delivers.*

The lesson here is that if a mother in labour feels safe and relaxed in her resting state, labour progresses well and delivery is more likely to happen as a natural process. If the mother becomes stressed, labour slows down and may stop completely. Stress however, during the second stage, speeds up delivery.

A mother needs a safe and familiar environment to aid the natural delivery of her baby, which is why some mothers and couples opt for a home birth. Ideally a hospital will meet this need too. Sometimes the unfamiliar and busy environment in a hospital may be perceived as a threat and the stress response triggers, slowing labour. Complications may then arise.

BIRTH, A KEY EVENT
There are key events in the life cycle of a human being. Birth is a key event. The others that occur in early life are conception and teething. Following a key event there is a significant shift in how we relate to life.

Birth is the transition from being within the mother to being outside of the mother. From that moment onwards the baby is using his/her lungs to breathe and feeding by swallowing milk.

From this new position outside the womb, a baby has a different relationship to his/her mother and father and they come into a closer relationship to the outside world. If the process of birth is straightforward, establishing these new relationships is natural. If birth is more complicated, the first experience of life may be too.

Conception is the initial key event, the coming into physical being. Teething is another time of transition.

A newborn baby's face structure and nervous system are set up for one main function, sucking, and this forms the basis of their early relationship to life. Teething may begin when only months old, but becomes significant between the ages of 12 and 18 months.

As babies' teeth develop, their face and jaw change shape and for them the focus of life moves from sucking to chewing – the stage of weaning. For many infants for the first time their food source is no longer their mother. This shifts the infant into a different relationship with their mother, their family and the world itself. Behavioural difficulties, including anger, are common at this time as the infant adjusts to his/her new orientation in life.

BIRTH IS A JOURNEY
From the womb out into the world birth is a journey. With a natural birth the journey is through the birth canal. This passage through the birth canal is a significant

life event for the baby and like all of life's major achievements, it is the experience of the journey that is key.

> *Take the example of a mountaineer. They may spend years planning a climb and months in preparation. When they are ready, they go for it. For them, it is the facing and overcoming of challenges during the climb that is their experience, not just being on the summit. There would be no learning or sense of achievement in just being airlifted up the mountain. And so it is with babies and birth.*

We have evolved over millions of years to be born; we hold within us an innate sense of birth. The baby's body develops and is programmed for a vaginal delivery. Their mother's body is similarly programmed to give birth. The baby needs to feel they have been born, and the mother in turn needs to feel that she has given birth. There is, therefore, something about birth that needs to feel complete, both for the baby and the mother. A natural delivery provides this.

A baby denied a natural delivery, for whatever reason, may not feel as though he/she has fully arrived. In a similar way, a mother who has given birth by caesarean section, or while anaesthetised, may not feel that the process of giving birth has ended. Without a complete ending, both body and mind can be left disorientated, not knowing what is going on.

NATURAL DELIVERY IS A PHYSIOLOGICAL TRIGGER

Physiology is the study of how our bodies work. There is something very significant about how a natural delivery helps stimulate the healthy functioning of a baby's body in readiness for life outside of the womb.

Labour is a process of regular uterine muscle contractions and increasing compression. These forces exert a deep massaging effect on the baby's head and body as it descends into the birth canal and this is an important process in preparing the baby's physiology for life after birth.

When the baby emerges decompression and expansion occur and so the baby's body begins to open up again. This process of expansion stimulates the movements of the cranial bones and the circulation and tide-like movements of the cerebrospinal fluid (CSF). Expansion encourages cranial-sacral motion. This helps the baby to process and recover from any strains, stress, or trauma resulting from his/her birth.

At conception a similar physiological trigger to the baby's embryological development occurs. The fertilisation of the mother's egg (ovum) is a far more powerful event after a sperm has survived the journey up through the uterus and fallopian tubes than it is if fertilisation occurs in a laboratory.

INTERVENTIONS

EMERGENCY CAESARIAN
An emergency caesarean is carried out when concern has arisen during labour and it is considered necessary to get the baby out quickly, either for the child's potential survival, the mother's, or both. Already the baby will have experienced many hours of labour. The labour may not have progressed well and the baby may have become stuck. He/she is likely to be stressed and may have already tipped into trauma.

When the birth process has entered the second stage, removing the baby by caesarean section is more complicated because the child must be pulled back up through the birth canal. In difficult circumstances this may involve the use of forceps. Frequently babies that have endured forceps caesarean extraction are deeply traumatised by their experience and likely to be angry.

An emergency caesarean can upset the physiological balance of the mother's body and that of the baby. Although the baby is safely out, his/her body may still be expecting to be born. Similarly, the mother's body may still be expecting to give birth. Eventually it will dawn on their respective bodies that nothing more is going to happen. It may take many weeks for their physiology to settle down, and in some cases this does not happen – their birth processes remain incomplete. It is difficult for the physiology of the human body to function normally when a previous process is left unfinished.

An incomplete birth process can occur following the use of an epidural (an injection into the lower spine during labour to deaden the pain of childbirth). With an epidural the mother is numb from the waist down, so she may not experience the physical sensations of giving birth. Physically and mentally she may not fully realise that her baby is born.

When the birth process is incomplete the mother may not physically recover well from the birth. She may struggle to heal, to stay well and to meet the demands of her growing baby. Bonding issues can arise.

A baby with an incomplete birth process can struggle to get used to life and may have feeding and behavioural issues. They may cry excessively or scream. Both mothers and babies do benefit from therapeutic help to complete their birth experiences. For mothers this could be councelling and for mothers and babies, alternative therapies such as craniosacral therapy, cranial osteopathy or homeopathy.

ELECTIVE CAESARIAN SECTION

An elective caesarean section is a planned caesarean. The reasons for this option could be:

- The position of the placenta
- Twins
- Breech presentation
- A pre-existing medical condition
- Health concerns regarding the mother or baby

With an elective caesarean, the mother's body does not go into labour and her baby may not be engaged beforehand. This means there will be no compressive or mechanical strains to the baby's head and body, but he/she will miss out on the physiological stimulation of their passage through the birth canal. If the operation goes well, the baby is unlikely to be traumatised, but they may be disorientated, stressed, or even angry at being brought into the world so abruptly.

Case study 3: Emily was born by elective caesarean. Her mother says that she is an intense baby and often wakes at night, crying.

Assessing Emily reveals that she has an active stress response in her nervous system. This is causing her chest to be tight and is affecting her breathing (sympathetic activation). Her stress response settles with one treatment and her chest and body relax. The following week her mother reports that Emily is much calmer and has been sleeping better.

FORCEPS DELIVERY

Forceps are a pincer-like medical instrument used to assist the delivery of the baby's head during the second stage. They make contact with both sides of the baby's head and some force may be applied to grasp the head and to guide and pull the baby out.

Before forceps are used, the baby may already have experienced a long and difficult labour. Commonly he/she is already stressed and may be in foetal distress. The addition of forceps can tip a baby into trauma. Contact points of the forceps on the baby's head can cause acute pain, bruising and sometimes cuts.

Babies who have had a forceps delivery are quite likely to have mechanical strains about their head and body. Frequently they experience pain, have an active stress response, or are in trauma. Forceps babies are commonly unsettled, have sleep, feeding, digestive and behavioural issues, cry excessively, or scream. A forceps baby is frequently an angry baby.

VENTOUSE DELIVERY

A ventouse is a suction cup attached to the baby's head to help pull him/her out during delivery. Like the use of forceps, by the time a ventouse is used the baby may have already endured a long and difficult labour, be stressed or be in trauma mode. The ventouse delivery may complicate this picture.

The effect of the ventouse on the baby's head is to stretch the dural membranes, brain and cranial bones. This can result in a cone-shaped head. The severity of the cone usually diminishes quickly as the baby's head settles after birth, but may not go entirely. Without appropriate cranial treatment the skull and dural membranes may remain tight and strained. This could cause the baby to be over-sensitive, reactive and tense, and to have trouble letting go. The symptoms of a ventouse baby also depend on what else happened during the birth in terms of mechanical strains, stress and trauma.

Case study 4: *Rosie was three weeks old when her mother brought her along. Her chief complaint was trapped wind and her daughter being unsettled. On questioning Rosie's mother she explained that Rosie also suffers from colic, frequently comfort feeds, is fractious, unable to lie on her back, makes poor eye contact and can get angry. Rosie had gone into foetal distress during her birth, passed meconium (baby's first poo) and was eventually delivered by ventouse, which left both her head and eyes bruised.*

> *The cranial therapy assessment showed that Rosie was stressed and very unsettled. She had marked strain of her left neck and upper back, cranial and spinal dural strain from late in the second stage which was still causing her pain (affect of the ventouse), and tight left temporal bone and frontal bone.*
>
> *Rosie had four cranial therapy treatments over six weeks. Her stress response quickly settled, as did the mechanical strain in her upper back and neck. It took the four sessions for her cranial and spinal dural membranes and her cranial bones to release well and soften.*
>
> *At the end of Rosie's treatment her mother reported that she is now settled, happy, very sociable and aware. She feeds well, has no colic, no anger, settles herself to sleep and sleeps all night.*

THE PREMATURE BABY

Premature babies are a special case. They have unique challenges due to their early arrival. When compared to an average baby, a premature baby is more likely to have issues with his/her organs and special senses, to have bonding issues and to have had medical intervention. To survive, the majority will have been triggered into the trauma response. This combination of factors leads to many premature babies having a higher level of need or dependency.

ORGANS AND SPECIAL SENSES
At a physiological level, a premature baby's organs and

special senses are not yet prepared for life outside the womb. Their lungs are not designed to breathe yet, stomach and intestines are not fully prepared for digestion, or the kidneys for elimination of waste products. However, in most premature babies the organs manage surprisingly well.

The premature baby's immature brain and special senses are hypersensitive to light and sound, and their body to touch. Their brain may be unable to process information well, or to filter out excessive sensory stimulation. This is not helped by the light, noise and bustle often present in neonatal units. Because their brain is unable to cope with this barrage of sensory information, it easily becomes over-whelmed, and triggers into stress, then trauma. The baby's developing mind frantically tries to comprehend his/her situation but frequently fails too. Often they have no peace.

The immature skull of a premature baby is soft and can easily deform or flatten while they are lying down in the incubator due to the weight of their head and the effect of gravity. This is why their body and head position is regularly changed by the nursing staff.

DEVELOPMENTAL ISSUES AND PREMATURE BABIES
As a premature baby grows and develops he/she is more likely to show movement, learning and behavioural

disorders if compared to a full-term baby. There are four main considerations for this:

- early learnt responses
- sensory processing disorders
- trauma
- brain damage

The premature baby's brain becomes programmed by his/her early life experience and this forms their reality (known as imprinting). Their brain learns to accept the struggle to survive, being alone in the incubator, the noises of the machines in the neonatal unit and regular medical interventions. A premature baby may struggle to cope with anything different because this has become their norm. Initially, once home, their brain may not cope well with the new environment because it is neurologically unfamiliar. Because of this early imprinting, they may demand a routine too.

Many premature babies remain hypersensitive throughout their life and/or continue to have sensory processing issues. It is helpful if their parents and later their carers and teachers have an appreciation of this; otherwise they can continually become overwhelmed and may have a tendency to cry excessively or even withdraw.

HOW YOUR BABY EMERGED INTO THE WORLD

The majority of premature babies drop into the trauma mode during their time spent in an incubator. Together with their strength of character, this is how they survive. In many of these babies their symptom and behaviour patterns are due to trauma. These may include: excessive crying and screaming, unresponsiveness, poor eye contact, detachment, sleep disturbances, hypervigilance and bonding issues. Repetitive medical interventions may continually re-traumatise the baby.

It is an unfortunate reality that some premature babies suffer a degree of brain damage as a result of their prematurity and early life experience. This may result in cerebral palsy, or other movement and learning disorders.

In assessing a premature baby it is important to differentiate between behaviours and disorders that are permanent due to brain damage, and those due to trauma that are potentially reversible. The baby and their family can then be directed to the most appropriate therapies.

Despite their early difficulties, some premature babies go on to become achievers. Surviving prematurity can help to create strength of character. Someone who has faced and overcome death at such an early age may have no fear about getting on with living.

PREMATURE BABIES AND TOUCH

Bonding presents challenges for a premature baby and his/her family. Because they are likely to spend the first part of their life in an incubator and are tube fed, there is little natural opportunity for touch. Initially touch may be limited to a parent being able to hold a hand or foot. This is extremely valuable. As development progresses, parents are able to hold and cuddle their baby for longer periods of time. Later, some go on to full breastfeeding. Talking gently and singing are soothing and also help the baby bond with his/her parents. Even just being there is a reassurance.

The key to being able to help a baby who has been traumatised, whether premature or full-term, is healthy human touch, especially skin contact. A newborn's body and nervous system is sensitive and receptive to touch; this is a primal function. They need to feel safe. Their brain learns to recognise and accept pleasant touch (pleasure) over pain. Pleasurable touch becomes calming and creates the sensation of safety. It is this felt sensation of safety that helps bring a baby out of trauma – feeling safe is our primary need.

***Case study 5:** There is the well-known story of a newborn who was pronounced dead and was covered up and laid aside for a couple of hours. The baby's mother, beginning to face her grief, asked to hold her baby and* *she was allowed to place his naked body on her bare chest. There he remained.*

A while later, he began to move; his heart had restarted and he was breathing. He continued to progress and made a full recovery. Perhaps he was in the freeze state of trauma? This event led to the development of 'Kangeroo Care', where premature babies remain placed on their mother's chest with skin contact, rather than being in an incubator.

DYLAN'S STORY

Dylan was born at six months of gestation. He is a twin, his sister, Ylaria, died. His breathing and oxygen levels were very erratic, his heart rate uncontrolled; he was struggling to survive. Against the advice of the neonatal staff, his devoted parents maintained a constant vigil by his incubator.

Assessing him at the age of one month in the intensive care neonatal unit, Dylan was deeply stressed. He was experiencing gagging and burning pain in his throat from his feeding tube, he had pain within his chest and his lungs were tight and failing to get enough oxygen, as was his brain. Dylan struggled to be mentally present. He was completely disorientated, his mind dissociating because it could not cope with his experience.

With regular craniosacral therapy over many weeks, Dylan's stress response calmed down, as did his heart and lungs. His throat relaxed and he became able to suck. Dylan was more settled and more present, despite having an ongoing issue with breathing and oxygenation. When his naso-gastric tube came out he went on to full breastfeeding.

When he first arrived home seven months later, Dylan became distraught – his brain could not cope with the unfamiliar environment of home. It took him many weeks to adjust. His brain had to relearn to accommodate change, even change for the better.

Dylan's mother Emma writes: As Dylan's parents we were thrown into a very traumatic situation in which one of our babies had died and her twin, Dylan, was critically ill for a long time. We had zero support from the medical profession regarding holistic care for Dylan, so independently we asked Peter to begin craniosacral therapy with him.

The beneficial effect was immediately clear. Dylan was calmer and more stable; his breathing was easier. He was able to relax more and to get a sense of himself and those around him. As time went on, Dylan became more content within himself, despite the traumas he experienced.

Once home over six months later, he needed further

treatments and now he is a very joyous soul indeed, even in the face of his challenges. Dylan would not be the child he is today without craniosacral therapy.

SOME POSTNATAL ISSUES

CUTTING OF THE CORD
The cutting of the umbilical cord is a procedure that is not given much significance. It is something that happens with every newborn and is frequently carried out immediately after birth. The cord is clamped and cut so that the baby can be handed to his/her mother, or taken away to be cleaned up, or assessed. There may be an acute medical need to do this, especially if the baby needs resuscitating. However, in many instances there is no immediate need to cut the cord and it may be disadvantageous to the newborn to do so. Most umbilical cords are long enough for the baby to be put to the breast after birth without the need to cut them.

If the cord is not cut immediately, it will continue to pulsate and supply the baby with blood from the placenta for another 20 to 40 minutes, even after the child has begun to breathe naturally. The cord naturally contracts and this is the ideal time to cut it. Leaving the cord to pulsate continues to enrich the baby's body with blood and oxygen. It is becoming a more common medical practice not to cut the cord immediately.

There is a condition known as 'cord shock'. If a baby's umbilical cord is cut quickly and before it has stopped pulsating the umbilical area may tense up due to shock. This causes a local trauma reaction. The umbilical tension may remain in the baby's abdomen and cause or contribute to digestive issues. Releasing this umbilical shock may help settle the digestive system of a baby.

BONDING

Bonding is the instinctive maternal and paternal link that exists between mother and baby, and father and baby. There is an innate feeling of togetherness, of closeness, of oneness.

Ideally bonding begins in the womb. It is enhanced during pregnancy and if all goes well, continues throughout life. Early bonding may be affected by the nature of the baby's conception and later by their parents' thoughts and feelings about the pregnancy and their developing baby. Circumstances and events during the pregnancy can affect the ability to bond, such as having to move house, the break-up of the relationship, a close bereavement, the mother being ill, having to take medication, threatened miscarriage, and a previous miscarriage, termination, or infant death.

Bonding issues can develop after the birth. If either the mother or her baby is traumatised by the birth

HOW YOUR BABY EMERGED INTO THE WORLD

experience, they may become withdrawn and this can affect their ability to bond well. This is likely to involve the social engagement response.

Separation of the baby from their mother after birth may also affect bonding. Babies have awareness of their environment from conception onwards so having spent nine months physically within their mother they do instinctively know when they are separated. A baby may be separated from his/her parents because of a medical issue, following baby surgery or having to spend time in an incubator. Of course adoption of a baby also affects bonding.

A caesarean delivery sometimes creates a bonding issue due to the incompleteness of the birthing process. The baby may not feel that he/she has been born; their mother may not feel that she has given birth. This situation is complicated by the use of anaesthetics; it also applies in a natural delivery when an epidural has been used.

If there is a problem bonding with their baby, a parent may not feel an emotional or physical connection with them. The joy of having a baby and caring for him/her may not be there. It is important for parents to recognise and acknowledge if there is a bonding issue, to know that it is not unusual and to seek appropriate help and support.

BABY SURGERY

One challenging area faced by some parents is that of baby surgery. Some babies need surgery immediately after birth to ensure their survival; others may do so at an early age. This may be traumatic for both the baby and his/her parents.

Most people who have surgery, whether as a baby or an adult, trigger into the trauma response to ensure their survival. An odd situation can develop after surgery because the person may feel OK but his/her body is still in the trauma response.

When a baby is anaesthetised before surgery he/she becomes unconscious. They are no longer awake to what happens during the surgery and so consciously they have no memory of it. However, their primitive nervous system (the brain stem) and unconscious mind experience all that happens during the surgery and react to this by going into trauma.

After surgery the baby's brain has no conscious recollection of what went on, yet his/her body and unconscious mind remembers. This creates a separation between their mind and body experience and between their conscious and unconscious mind. This is one reason why babies and children may develop night terrors, behavioural disturbances, a lack of confidence or fears and anxiety, following a surgical procedure: they are unconsciously reacting to something traumatic that happened of which they have no conscious memory. Night terrors in babies and children are also commonly linked to traumatic events in their birth process for the same reason.

Receiving craniosacral therapy after surgery can help a baby's body process the state of trauma so that his/her mind and body responses become integrated once again.

POSTNATAL DEPRESSION
A common finding in women who have postnatal depression is that they have not yet got over the experience of giving birth. This is as much an issue of the physiology of the body as it is of the mind.

After giving birth a mother's body begins the process of recovery and repair. This process is a function of her parasympathetic nervous system and occurs when the body is in the resting mode. If a mother remains stressed, physically injured or traumatised after the birth of her baby, repair and recovery may not happen completely and she may fail to get over the birth. Postnatal depression then has a greater tendency to develop.

Coping with the daily needs of the newborn creates further stress, especially if the baby is unsettled. There may come a point when the mother and her body no longer cope. This may show as poor wound healing, physical and mental exhaustion, bonding issues and later depression.

It is of great benefit for a mother to receive craniosacral therapy or cranial osteopathy after giving birth to help her body release the stress and trauma responses from the birth process and to aid her recovery. A mother is then in a better position to be present for her baby and meet his/her ongoing needs. Many cranial therapists prefer to work with mother and baby together for this reason; it also helps with bonding issues.

Chapter 5.

HOW YOUR BABY CAN BE HELPED

To be able to help a baby, particularly one who cries excessively or screams, the child needs a therapeutic approach which is safe, gentle and supportive, acknowledges who they are, is able to assess accurately what is going on and makes a positive difference. Today such a therapy exists and it is known by two different names:

1. craniosacral therapy
2. cranial osteopathy

For the purpose of simplicity, craniosacral therapy and cranial osteopathy will be referred to jointly as 'cranial therapy'; they are principally the same therapy. Someone who practises cranial therapy will be described as a cranial therapist.

This chapter explores the nature of cranial therapy – what it is, the science behind it, and how it works. It also considers those times when it does not appear to work, or does not work.

WHAT IS CRANIAL THERAPY?

THE HISTORY OF CRANIAL THERAPY
Both craniosacral therapy and cranial osteopathy are based in the original teachings of Dr Andrew Taylor Still (1828–1917), the founder of osteopathy and Dr William Garner Sutherland (1873–1954), the founder of cranial osteopathy and a pupil of Dr Still. Both of these men were American, medical doctors and osteopaths. In America osteopathy is taught as a speciality of medicine, so an American osteopath may practise surgery, osteopathy and prescribe medication.

Dr Sutherland was an anatomist – he studied the human bones. One day, while studying the bones of the skull and their sutures (joints), he had the insight that the sutures seemed to be designed for movement. Dr Sutherland realised that all the skull bones fit together in a way that allows the skull to expand and contract very slightly in a particular pattern. He put this theory into practice by making a helmet that selectively locked up his skull bones. When he wore this helmet, not only did he develop symptoms in his head, but also in his body and with his organs. He had stumbled across cranial-sacral motion, the subtle pattern of movement of our bones, tissues and fluids. From his discoveries Dr Sutherland developed the field of cranial osteopathy.

It was later, in the 1970s, that another American osteopath and surgeon, Dr John Upledger, first coined the term 'craniosacral therapy'. Dr Upledger, through his teaching and writing, was responsible for bringing craniosacral therapy into the public domain. He founded the Upledger Institute and began training other types of healthcare professionals and interested members of the public in craniosacral therapy.

Cranial therapy continues to advance today under both practices of cranial osteopathy and craniosacral therapy.

CRANIAL THERAPY USES THE SENSE OF TOUCH
Cranial therapy is a hands-on therapy based in the skilful use of touch – one of our special senses. We have touch sensors (proprioceptors) all over our skin, but with a particularly high concentration on our hands and fingers. One of the main reasons why we have evolved so well as a species is because of the dexterity and

sensitivity of our hands. This has enabled us to understand and manipulate our environment and create: our hands are the tools that have shaped our world.

All of our senses can be trained to a high degree. A musician has a highly developed sense of hearing, of tone. A chef has a highly developed sense of taste and smell. Our sense of touch can be developed in many different ways – the potter, the carpenter, the artist, the osteopath.

Take the example of Braille. Have you ever tried to read Braille? If you were given a sheet of paper with Braille on it, the chances are that all you would feel is a whole lot of dots. For you they would have no significance but for a blind person this is their written language. They have developed their sense of touch to the degree that these dots can be translated into letters, words and speech.

And so it is with cranial therapy. With skilled training a cranial therapist develops his/her sense of touch to the degree that he/she can feel, read, what is going on in the human body. He/she can feel where bones have tightened, tissues have twisted, and where stress or trauma is held. A cranial therapist can feel the subtle movement pattern of cranial-sacral motion.

MOVEMENT IS LIFE

Movement is life – everything in nature moves. In the natural world there are the rays of the sun, the opening of flowers, the blowing of the wind, the flowing of rivers and streams, and the sliding of tectonic plates.

As human beings, like other animals, even when we are at rest, our bodies are never completely still, unless we are dead. Our cells jostle around, fluids transfer in and out of the cell walls, our heart beats, blood circulates, our chest and lungs expand and contract with breathing, stomach and intestines digest, our brain receives and processes information, thoughts come and go and there is cranial-sacral motion. Where there is life there is movement; where there is free movement there is health.

A cranial therapist uses his/her trained sense of touch to evaluate the subtle movement patterns of the human body that we cannot see. If you place your hands on your own chest you may feel the beat of your heart and the movement of your breathing. A cranial therapist is also trained to feel cranial-sacral motion. Cranial-sacral motion is the rhythmic expansion and contraction of all our body tissues, including the bones of our skull. It is the sensing, evaluation and treatment of this motion pattern that is cranial therapy.

WHOLENESS

The title 'cranial' therapy is misleading because it is not just a treatment for the head, the cranium. Cranial therapy is a treatment approach for the whole body and the whole person.

During birth it is not just your baby's head and body that are born, they are born too. Your baby experiences his/her birth. The wholeness of birth also includes their mother, father, whoever else was present and the environment where the birth took place.

Wholeness is not an idea; it is an experience. We can experience ourselves as whole. If we are not whole, we must be functioning as separate parts. We may use expressions like: my body is disjointed, my leg feels like it does not belong to me, my life has fallen apart. We may also say, 'I feel complete, in harmony, in tune with my body, whole'.

Because being whole is a physical experience it is possible to sense wholeness with touch. One of the things a cranial therapist is trained to do is to sense the state of wholeness in an individual. When a cranial therapist places his/her hands on a client's body, they can assess that person for their state of wholeness. Wholeness can be felt from anywhere in the body. When assessing a problematic part of the body, that part is always understood in relation to the rest of the body as a whole.

We only heal when we are whole. A part of the body will only get fully better if it has an established relationship with the whole of the body. This is why orthodox medicine can fail to help people, because it treats the human body as separate parts. Drugs and surgery do nothing to promote wholeness. Restoring wholeness is an essential part of any healing process. If the sense of wholeness is restored in a baby, he/she will begin to get better.

Cranial therapy is a hands-on therapeutic approach, which uses the highly developed sense of touch of the therapist to assess and treat clients by encouraging and restoring wholeness and the natural expression of cranial-sacral motion throughout the body.

CRANIAL THERAPY, ANATOMY IN MOTION

LIVING ANATOMY
Cranial therapy is based in the medical science of anatomy. To become a cranial therapist you study anatomy. One of the main differences between orthodox medicine and cranial therapy is in how anatomy is taught and understood.

Historically, orthodox medicine was based on the study of dead bodies. Even today, medical students do dissections. Dead bodies are cold, hard and motionless – lifeless. The study of dead anatomy gives the student an idea of the different tissues and organs that make up the human body and where they are located.

In contrast, cranial therapists learn anatomy by practicing with live people as well as studying. A living body is warm and soft and expresses movement, vitality, wholeness and its uniqueness. All these qualities are perceptible with touch.

Using their developing sense of touch and by placing their hands in different locations on the body, cranial therapy students learn to experience and understand the anatomy of the human body and how it works. They learn how the different tissues of the body feel, how they move, how they relate to each other and how they relate to the whole: bones, joints, muscles, fasciae, nerves, brain, organs and fluids. Fasciae are the thin, continuous sheets of fibrous tissue that hold the body together, sometimes referred to as 'sinew'.

As training develops, it becomes possible for the cranial therapy student to sense with touch the movement of the cranial bones, the tension pattern of the dural membranes, the rhythmic expansion and contraction of the brain, the tide-like movements of the cerebrospinal fluid, the expression of cranial-sacral motion and the interconnectedness of the whole body. Anatomy is a living science.

As a cranial therapist gains experience working with the living anatomy of healthy individuals, he/she also develops an awareness of when something is not right. With practise it becomes possible to feel patterns of mechanical compression and strain in a adult's or baby's body; the active stress response, held emotional states of grief and anger, the trauma response and the sensory processing ability of the brain. Learning to touch and understand living anatomy becomes a process of whole body assessment. Assessment naturally progresses to treatment.

OCTOPUS OUT OF WATER
For anyone who studies medical sciences such as biology, anatomy, physiology and embryology, it becomes difficult not to believe in the process of evolution. Evolution explains so much about how the human body develops and how it works.

The essential part of a human being is their central nervous system. If you picture the shape of your brain and spinal cord, it is a lot like an octopus – the brain is like the head of the octopus and the spinal cord and nerves dangling behind are its legs. The brain and spinal cord are surrounded by fluid, which is enclosed by the tissues and bones of the spine and skull. This CSF (cerebrospinal fluid) is equivalent to the sea. The rest of our body, torso, arms and legs carry the octopus around on dry land and enable it to explore, chase and catch prey and escape from predators. Evolutionarily, a human being is like an octopus out of water. Essentially we are a brain and spinal cord floating around in a bit of residual sea, contained by our dural membranes and bones, and carried around in a body on land.

To complete this story, in the same way that the sea is characterised by waves and tides, the fluid surrounding the central nervous system, the CSF, constantly moves in a tide-like manner. Cranial-sacral motion is equivalent to the ebb and flow of the sea. We are all waves arising from the same ocean.

CRANIAL-SACRAL MOTION
Cranial-sacral motion is the subtle movement pattern of living tissue as was first recognised by Dr Sutherland. This is a pattern of regular and rhythmic expansion and contraction, like breathing. Sometimes it is called 'primary respiration' as opposed to secondary respiration, which is lung breathing. Some mystics and schools of cranial therapy call it 'The Breath of Life'.

HOW YOUR BABY CAN BE HELPED

This involuntary rhythmic movement pattern involves all our body tissues, our bones, joints, membranes, muscles, fasciae, ligaments, fluids, nervous system and organs. It is a whole body expression.

Cranial-sacral motion can be felt with trained hands anywhere on the body and occurs at different rates. These rates are described as rhythms or tides and there are three main ones: fast tide, slow or mid-tide and long tide.

The fast tide is technically called the cranial rhythmic impulse (CRI). This tide reflects what is going on at the surface of our body; it is like the waves on the surface of the sea. If we get over-excited, stressed or injured (sympathetic nervous system activation), this tide speeds up, either just local to an injury, or over the whole body. The fast tide behaves like the sea during a storm, although it may not slow completely once a storm has passed.

The slow or mid-tide is a deeper tide, and is more easily felt when we are calm and relaxed in our resting state. It is more of a function of our parasympathetic nervous system. With cranial therapy, being able to help the body slow down from the fast tide into the mid-tide calms down the stress response and can help begin to bring someone out of trauma.

The long tide is always present but is mainly felt and experienced in states of deep relaxation or connectedness, such as when we feel totally at one with ourselves and our surroundings: in the zone. It is also felt in moments of peak experience and is a profoundly healing state.

THE FIVE PHENOMENA
In order to convey his understanding of cranial osteopathy, Dr Sutherland recognised five key phenomena characterising cranial-sacral motion. They are:

1. **The articular mobility of the cranial bones.** The human skull is constructed of 21 bones, which are jointed together. These joints allow movement between adjacent bones, which in turn allows for the rhythmic expansion and contraction of the skull, brain and central nervous system.
2. **The reciprocal mobility of the cranial membranes.** The dural membranes lining the brain and spinal cord move in the pattern of expansion and contraction. Tension or a pull in one part of the dural membranes will simultaneously affect all the other parts.
3. **The inherent fluctuation of the cerebrospinal fluid (CSF).** The CSF physically circulates around the brain and spinal cord, but it also has an

inherent motion pattern expressing the three tides. Inherent means this movement occurs as a natural function of being alive. Our life force expresses itself as cranial-sacral motion.
4. **The inherent mobility of the central nervous system.** Our brain and spinal cord are mobile within the confines of the skull and spine and also inherently move in the expansion and contraction phases of cranial-sacral motion.
5. **Involuntary motion of the sacrum between the ilia.** The sacrum moves freely between the two sides of the pelvis (the left and right ilia). This movement is a key part of cranio-sacral motion and also involves the whole body structure. It is particularly linked with the movement of the spine and the cranial bones, but also to our ribs, arms, hands, legs and feet. Cranial-sacral motion involves every tissue that makes up the living anatomy of our body.

HOW CRANIAL THERAPY WORKS

Cranial therapy is a safe and gentle, hands-on approach to treating babies, children and adults. It uses a very light, still touch to listen to what each unique individual needs, to deepen the resting state and thereby encourage the processing and integration of past experience and to restore healthy cranial-sacral motion. Cranial therapy works by encouraging the innate healing and recovery response.

ENCOURAGING THE RECOVERY RESPONSE

Another survival system that has evolved in human beings is that of recovery. The recovery system involves repair, healing and maintenance.

Without an immune system we would die from the slightest infection. Without a repair system even the simplest skin cut or bone fracture would not heal. The human body is a self-healing and self-repairing organism; it constantly strives to maintain balance and health.

Health problems arise within the human body after something happens which is too sudden, or too intense to cope with, such as marked physical injury, stress or trauma. The body becomes overwhelmed, tries to get over the experience and if it fails, full recovery may not be possible. Patterns of symptoms then occur and in the longer term, health issues arise.

Recovery occurs optimally when we are relaxed or sleeping deeply – in situations in which the parasympathetic nervous system is in operation, the resting state. If we remain stressed, complete healing may not occur.

HOW YOUR BABY CAN BE HELPED

This is why a strained, stressed or traumatised baby is not able naturally to overcome their experience.

Adults with repetitive stress injuries (RSI) are usually stuck in the stress response, so their over-used muscles and tendons do not recover properly. This is also true of professional footballers – their bodies may never get adequate rest or recuperation from playing, so their injuries do not heal well and become ongoing.

Therapeutically it is possible to promote recovery by helping the client drop from the stress or trauma response into the resting state. This is one way in which cranial therapy begins to help babies who have not got over the experience of their birth; the gentle and safe touch of the cranial therapist creates a pleasant and unthreatening sensation in which the baby's body can begin to drop into the resting state and let go of the stress and trauma responses. The baby's body then begins to process and release the experiences causing the overwhelm; recovery becomes possible.

LISTENING TO THE BODY

The principal tools a cranial therapist uses are their hands and the sense of touch. If you watch a cranial therapist at work you will observe that they sit still and that their hands do not move on the client's body. Cranial therapy is not like massage; it does not involve strokes, pushing or pulling. There is a reason for this: you can feel more deeply into the body with your hands when they are still. Movement is a distraction. Take the example of a hunter:

A hunter is in the forest, tracking deer (to take photos). It is very difficult to see far ahead because of the density of trees and the twilight. If the hunter walked around, breaking twigs and calling out, the deer would disappear for miles around. When the hunter remains still and tunes into the forest with his senses, the deer are not threatened and he may sense where they are; they may even cross his path.

And so it is with cranial therapy, the listening touch. The cranial therapist takes a light, still hold, which may be anywhere on the baby's body (the touch is gentle because the therapist wishes to remain neutral). If the touch involves pressure, the baby's body may become threatened or stressed. With this light touch the baby's body may feel safe enough to reveal its experiences, its 'held tissue memory'. Helping the baby then becomes possible. The cranial-sacral touch is often described as the 'butterfly touch', the weight of a butterfly on the skin.

ENCOURAGING PROCESSING AND INTEGRATION
Most babies who cry excessively or scream have not got over the experience of their birth. If they can be helped

to get over their experiences, they can recover. Cranial therapy helps babies to process and integrate what has happened.

With a baby, their experience of birth is held as tissue memory within the body. This may be a pattern of mechanical strain, the stress response or the trauma response. Cranial therapists relate to these held patterns of tissue memory by using touch – the non-verbal communication.

By gently holding a baby with an unthreatening and neutral touch, the baby's body may feel safe enough to reveal to the cranial therapist what it is holding; its patterns of experience.

For example, the cranial therapist may sense this as a pattern of compression and strain about a baby's head and neck, they may sense that a baby is still stressed by the intensity and duration of labour, they may sense a baby could no longer cope with his/her experience and is detached due to trauma, or they may sense a baby is holding grief or anger. All this information is conveyed through the perceptive sense of the listening touch.

If the therapist is able to sense a held pattern of experience within a baby and they maintain their neutral and safe touch, something happens. The baby's body automatically directs itself to the held pattern and starts to process, work through, and integrate the previous experience. This is a function of the recovery system. Their body is constantly trying to reach a state of balance and health and embraces the help of the cranial therapist to make this possible. It is the listening touch that triggers this healing process, sometimes within seconds of making a hand contact.

The job of the cranial therapist is to maintain the safe and neutral listening touch, so that the baby's body continues to process, integrate and off-load past experience. The cranial therapist is a catalyst only; they create and hold the safe therapeutic space using touch, but they do not make the changes happen. Healing and recovery arise from the strength and intelligence within the baby's body.

This healing process takes time, patience and skill. It occurs one step at a time. This is why babies are recommended to have a series of treatments. Knowing how to help regulate this process and when to stop is another skill of the cranial therapist. If too much processing happens in one go, a baby may become overwhelmed and then upset.

As the baby releases his/her past experience, they become more settled, whole and complete. Their symptom patterns change. They may become calm, sleep better, cry less, stop screaming and digestion improves; they may become content for the first time. The baby's body can now put its energy into growing, developing and being social.

RESTORING CRANIAL-SACRAL MOTION
Cranial-sacral motion is how our life force expresses itself as a subtle rhythmic movement pattern of expansion and contraction in all our body tissues. In health this movement is free and expansive.

Where problems exist in the human body caused by injury, stress or trauma, restriction results and the easy, fluid movement of cranial-sacral motion becomes interrupted. Where bones are compressed or stuck, there is no motion. If tissues are twisted, the motion pattern is irregular. If a person is stressed, the motion pattern speeds up; if they are in trauma, the motion pattern may be absent.

When using the listening touch to sense the baby's whole body, the cranial therapist may also feel for the quality of cranial-sacral motion, how free and fluid it is. This enables them to gain an understanding of what is happening with the baby's bones, membranes, muscles, fasciae, nervous system, organs and fluids. The cranial therapist can then build up a picture of the health of a baby, how he/she has been affected by the birth process and why this is causing their symptoms now.

For example, if cranial-sacral motion is expressing as a twisting movement through a baby's neck, it is likely to indicate a neck strain. If cranial-sacral motion is jammed up around the skull, this may indicate head compression. If cranial-sacral motion is held about the umbilicus this may indicate cord-cutting shock. If cranial-sacral motion is speeded up in the whole body, it could indicate an active stress response. If cranial-sacral motion is absent, it could indicate past trauma.

In the same way that maintaining the safe and neutral listening touch triggers the response of processing and integration within a baby, it also triggers cranial sacral motion to want to become free and expressive. This results in expansion of compressive strains, unwinding of twisting strains, release of the stress response and integration back into the body following trauma. Sometimes with a baby you can see this happening: their body relaxes, they stop crying or screaming, their expression softens and they become peaceful. When the treatment is complete, cranial-sacral motion will express deeply throughout the whole body. Now the body is functioning normally and there is wholeness and health.

WHEN CRANIAL THERAPY FAILS TO HELP

The reality is that cranial therapy does not help every baby; it is not a cure-all. This section explores some common reasons why some babies appear not to respond well to cranial therapy, or do not respond well.

PERSEVERENCE
You will hear stories of crying babies who receive cranial therapy and are completely transformed after one session. This does happen and it is not rare, but please do not go along expecting this.

The main reason why a baby fails to get better with cranial therapy is because the parents have not persevered with the treatment for long enough. Some parents will try one or two treatments for their baby, but if they are not getting better at this stage, will decide it is not working and not continue. Stopping here is not great for your baby; his/her treatment process is only beginning.

If you consider that the average baby experiences 24 hours of labour and a further hour being delivered, possibly with intervention, all the stresses and strains of birth are not going to resolve in one or two 30-minute treatments. Cranial therapy is a process and it takes time.

Typically a baby will process and integrate a lot of his/her strain and stress issues in the first five sessions. However, it can still take five to six treatments to begin to help a baby very unsettled from birth, particularly one who cries excessively or screams. A premature baby may need in excess of 10 treatments.

If you consult a cranial therapist with your baby, please go along with the intention of having six sessions, even if they do not need them all. If after six treatments your baby is showing no signs of improvement, then you need to have a conversation with the therapist to discuss the benefits of continuing.

If your baby has had six treatments with a craniosacral therapist and they are not improving, it can be worth having a second opinion from a cranial osteopath and vice versa. This is because there can be slight differences in emphasis between the two approaches and your baby may respond better to one of them.

THE SKILL OF THE THERAPIST
The level of skill and experience of the cranial therapist may determine whether the treatment of a baby is successful. This particularly relates to complex cases. Generally, the longer a cranial therapist has been in practice and the more post-graduate trainings they have completed, the more effective their skills will be.

Your cranial therapist will usually admit if they are out of their depth treating your baby. In this situation they may recommend a more experienced colleague.

The skill for a cranial therapist when treating a baby is to keep a feather-light touch, to remain neutral and to give the baby space, not to overcrowd them. This is because birth, by its very nature, is a compressive process and the cranial therapist does not wish to intensify this. For this reason a cranial therapist will usually begin assessing and treating a baby by holding his/her feet or legs and not the head.

Should the cranial therapist inadvertently work too intensely or with too much hand pressure, the baby may react by becoming more stressed and more upset.

Most cranial therapists are very open people. If you have any concerns about your baby's progress, or lack of it, discuss this with them. You are never obliged to carry on with cranial therapy; it is your choice. If you decide to stop the treatment for any reason, do inform the cranial therapist of your decision.

SOMETIMES IT IS NOT ONLY ABOUT YOUR BABY

Sometimes it is not helpful to assume that if your baby is crying excessively or screaming it is just about them. This could be true, but their environment is an important factor too. If either one, or both parents, are stressed or traumatised from the birth process, this could have an adverse effect on their baby. The home or hospital environment and the behaviour of other family members are all influences that can affect a baby and how effectively he/she responds to cranial therapy.

Following treatment from a cranial therapist, if a baby is living in a situation that is noisy, unsettled or stressful, they may feel unsafe and not process the effects of their treatment well.

Your baby's primary need is to feel safe and to know you are there. This is why co-sleeping or sleeping in the same room can be essential for a young baby. A baby who develops security within his/her own body will enjoy their own room when they are ready.

You may wish as a parent to consider whether you would like to have cranial therapy too. It can be particularly beneficial to mothers to have a series of cranial therapy sessions to help recuperation from any sense of strain, intervention, surgery, stress or trauma residual from giving birth. Some cranial therapists prefer to work with the mother and baby together. Every member of a family may benefit from being able to talk about, process and complete their experience of your baby's birth.

HOW YOUR BABY CAN BE HELPED

AN OUTSTANDING MEDICAL ISSUE

A baby who fails to respond well to cranial therapy and continues to cry excessively or scream may have an undiagnosed medical condition without anyone having realised this so far. It is not the role of the cranial therapist to medically diagnose your baby. This is why it is important for you to consult your doctor about any concerns you may have with your baby.

If a cranial therapist is treating a baby and the baby is responding well to the treatment, but their symptoms are not changing, the therapist will need to consider if the child has other issues. Examples of this are milk or lactose intolerance, severe reflux, unexplained pain, or a sensory processing issue. In these situations going back to your doctor, or being referred to a paediatrician, are advisable.

If your baby is crying excessively or screaming and is not getting better despite having a series of cranial therapy treatments, you have several options. To persevere with the treatment a little longer, go for a second opinion with a different cranial therapist, consider whether there are any issues in your environment that may be contributing to your baby's upset, or to return to your doctor for further advice or investigation.

Chapter 6
TAKING YOUR BABY TO A CRANIAL THERAPIST

If your baby is crying excessively, screaming, or has other issues that concern you as a parent, you can try cranial therapy. This chapter looks at how to find a cranial therapist, what happens when your baby has an appointment, what happens during the treatment, and what to expect afterwards.

It takes several years of training and supervised clinical experience for a cranial therapist to work safely and effectively with babies and children. The descriptions contained in this chapter are for your understanding only; this is not a self-help instruction manual. If you become interested in practicing cranial therapy, professional training is available.

TAKING YOUR BABY TO A CRANIAL THERAPIST

PREPARING FOR AN APPOINTMENT

HOW TO FIND A CRANIAL THERAPIST
All cranial therapists are registered and insured with a professional association. If you do not know of a cranial therapist who treats babies, the best way to find one is by personal recommendation. Ask other mothers if they have had any of their babies or children treated. Failing this, ask your friends, colleagues, or health professionals such your midwife, health visitor, active birth teacher, or an alternative health practitioner.

If you are unable to locate a cranial therapist through personal contact, the next best option is to do an internet search. Enter craniosacral therapy or cranial osteopathy and your hometown into a search engine. This will come up with some options. Not all craniosacral therapists and cranial osteopaths treat babies, so you will need to check their websites for details, or phone and ask.

If you prefer to go through a professional register, most advancing countries have associations of craniosacral therapists and osteopaths. Each association will have a directory of registered members, which you can also search for on the internet. (YOUR NEXT STEP includes the website addresses of the main cranial therapy associations in the UK and some world-wide suggestions).

A word of advice when choosing a cranial therapist: do pick someone local, ideally within 10 miles (16 kilometres). It is not good for your baby to spend a long time travelling in a car before and after an appointment and if you need to return on several occasions it becomes impractical, exhausting and easy to give up on.

Some mothers travel hundreds of miles to see a cranial therapist recommended by a friend; this is rarely necessary. The only time this may be important is if your baby is proving difficult to treat, or has a rare condition and you have been recommended to someone with specialist knowledge and experience a greater distance away.

Cranial therapists make appointments by telephone, text or e-mail. Most have their own website with their practice and contact details.

SOME PRACTICALITIES
A baby can be treated by a cranial therapist at any age, even just after delivery. Indeed the earlier the better, but it is never too late. Some mothers routinely bring a newborn to their cranial therapist for a check-up. A

TAKING YOUR BABY TO A CRANIAL THERAPIST

baby does not have to have something wrong, though most are brought along because of excessive crying, screaming, digestive issues or poor sleep.

Many couples who decide to try cranial therapy go along together with their baby, particularly to the first appointment. This is great and is to be recommended. It is important for both parents to be comfortable with cranial therapy and the therapist.

If cranial therapy is new to you and the baby's father is unable or unwilling to attend, it is fine to go along with a relative or friend for support. Other people are usually curious about cranial therapy and it is interesting to watch.

Your baby will remain clothed at all times because cranial therapists are able to feel through your child's clothes and nappy. It is common for a baby to get hotter during a cranial treatment as his/her body responds. If this happens and they become unsettled you may need to remove a layer.

If your baby is fed before the session, they are less likely to become upset during the treatment because of hunger. Should he/she become obviously hungry during a treatment session, it is OK to stop and feed them if you are comfortable with this. In fact this may help the session. Cranial therapists are experienced at working around you and your baby's needs.

You will need to ask the cranial therapist how much he/she charges. The cost of a cranial therapy session for a baby is typically less than for an adult because cranial therapists like to make this work accessible to as many babies and families as possible. Cranial therapists may also make an extra allowance for parents on low incomes. Some big cities have low-cost clinics for babies and children. An appointment will last from between 30 and 60 minutes depending on how the cranial therapist works. If you are unsure whether cranial therapy will help your baby, discuss your concerns with a cranial therapist by telephone before committing to an appointment.

A HEALTHY CHALLENGE TO YOUR MIND
Cranial therapy is unlike most other forms of treatment because the cranial therapist's hands remain unmoving on your baby's body during the assessment and the treatment. While maintaining this still contact, the therapist may be able to describe to you how your baby is feeling now, what he/she has experienced and why this is upsetting them.

This may challenge your mind because often we are used to treatments involving obvious effort and action.

TAKING YOUR BABY TO A CRANIAL THERAPIST

You are likely to wonder what the cranial therapist is doing, how they can tell you what is happening and how continuing to hold your baby could possibly help.

Our brain has two cerebral hemispheres, right and left. The right side of the brain is the side used for creativity and perception, the left side is used for logical thinking. Cranial therapists are trained to use both sides of their brain when they are working. Much of their understanding of your baby comes from their perception of touch and how this is processed by their right brain; they are not working things out logically.

As the parent watching, it is the left side of your brain that will try to work out what the cranial therapist is doing and you may become confused. Just go with this. If you are able to settle into your feeling self, you may also perceive what the therapist senses. Some parents are already instinctively linked into their baby this way.

Most cranial therapists will explain what they are doing and why, but you can always ask about anything you are concerned about or perplexed by. Cranial therapy may be a healthy challenge to your mind and it is an education.

CRANIAL THERAPY AND ORTHODOX MEDICINE
Most medical professionals do not know enough about

cranial therapy and for this reason are unable to recommend it. In general, doctors do not refer babies to cranial therapists; it is not part of their remit.

You do not have to get your doctor's permission to consult a cranial therapist; they work independently to other health services and it is your free choice to do so. However, if you have a health concern about your baby, it is always advisable to consult your doctor first.

Many health visitors and midwives recommend taking crying or screaming babies to see a cranial therapist because they experience at first hand the relief this therapy frequently brings.

It is possible for a cranial therapist to work in a neonatal unit if they are asked to do so by a parent, provided they get permission from the ward staff nurse at each visit.

ASSESSING YOUR BABY

The assessment of your baby is a process that includes taking the case history, an examination, discussion of findings and asking for consent before moving into the treatment phase.

THE CASE HISTORY
Like all medical appointments, the first thing that

happens when you visit a cranial therapist is that they take the case history. This gives you (and your partner) the opportunity to tell your story about the pregnancy, the birth and what has happened since. This is important and is the first step in the therapeutic process. Just talking about what has happened can begin to make a difference.

The initial question you will be asked is, 'How can I help you?' or 'What is your main concern?' It is important for the cranial therapist to recognise the key issue that concerns you about your baby. This is known as the 'Chief Complaint'. Your chief complaint could be that your baby cries excessively, screams, or is inconsolable. The cranial therapist's intention is always to make a difference to the chief complaint where possible.

Next, you will be asked about your experience of your baby's birth – what happened and how you managed. This includes how labour started, how it progressed, how long it was, when you may have gone to hospital, how easily you dilated, your baby's position, use of painkillers, the nature of the delivery, any interventions or foetal distress and how you and your baby were after delivery. You may also be asked about your pregnancy and any issues that arose during that period.

The cranial therapist will ask questions about what has happened to you and your baby since the birth, how you both are now and any concerns you may have. For example:

- Has your baby had any serious illness, injections, or hospital visits?
- Is your baby sociable, able to make eye contact and developing OK?
- Is your baby happy, content, feeding well and gaining weight?
- Does your baby experience feeding, breathing, or sleeping issues, or problems with wind or digestion?
- Can your baby be laid down or is he/she only settled while you are holding them?
- Is your baby unsettled, crying, screaming, in pain, or angry?
- Is your baby full-on and having difficulty letting go?

Two other common questions are:

- What do you understand about cranial therapy?
- What are your expectations from the treatment?

You are welcome to ask the cranial therapist questions too.

TAKING YOUR BABY TO A CRANIAL THERAPIST

THE ASSESSMENT
Taking the case history gives the cranial therapist the background to what your baby has experienced, but to gain more information, he/she needs to be assessed. The assessment is where the cranial therapist uses their perceptive skills to establish what is going on with your baby, why they are upset and how to begin helping them. This involves both a visual and touch assessment.

Observing your baby can reveal how they are. Do they appear calm, or upset? If they are upset, how are they crying – moaning gently, crying inconsolably or screaming as if in pain? It is totally OK to turn up to an appointment with your baby crying inconsolably. Indeed this is not unusual – they don't have to be calm to be assessed or treated.

A visual assessment will also show if your baby is comfortable in his/her body or whether they are tense, straining and struggle to keep still. Their facial expressions and ability to make and maintain social contact are noticed too.

The next part of the assessment uses the listening touch. Normally a young baby will remain held by you or sat on your lap, whichever is the easiest position for you both. An older or contented baby may be OK lying on a treatment couch. If your baby is asleep in a pram or car seat, the assessment can be done from there. The cranial therapist makes a gentle hand contact on your baby's body.

Hand contact is first made with a more neutral part of your baby's body such as one or both feet or legs, or with your baby's back or pelvis. Making initial contact with the head can be too much for them and they may get overwhelmed and cry.

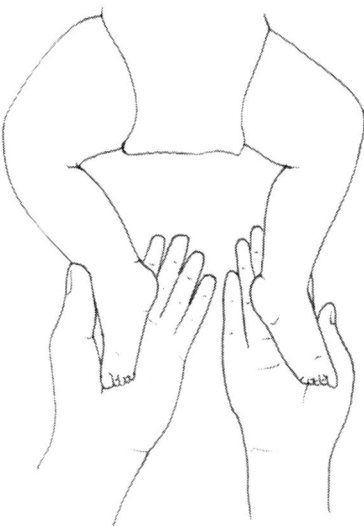

Figure 4. The cranial therapy hand hold on a baby's legs.

With the listening touch the therapist is open to perceiving a general impression from your baby's body about how he/she is now and how best to help them. Such impressions can include:

- the sense that they have not got over the experience of their birth
- a sense of overwhelm and not being able to cope
- disorientation and over-sensitive eyes
- a sensory processing difficulty
- being physically tense, twisted, or compressed and being able to identify the specific location of the strain and which tissues are involved
- the quality of expression of cranial-sacral motion and where it is being restricted
- a sense that your baby is experiencing pain
- an active stress response, with a very tense body and hyper-vigilant nervous system
- a feeling of absence as though they are not fully present in their body
- a need to be held and supported
- a lack of wholeness and integration
- a sense of complete ease, contentment and peace

After the assessment, the cranial therapist will discuss his/her findings with you and may be able to explain the reasons why your baby cries excessively or screams. They will also say if they think they can help you and your baby, how many sessions your baby may need and what may happen during the course of the treatment. Your verbal consent is then needed before progressing to the treatment phase.

CONSENT
Giving consent is giving permission. The cranial therapist should stop after an assessment and ask you if you consent to them treating your baby. This is a legal obligation. As the parent, you have the right to say no. Usually this is verbal consent. Less commonly, a cranial therapist will ask for written consent. In this case they will have a form for you to sign, which states that you agree to have your baby treated.

If you have no previous knowledge or experience of cranial therapy and the treatment of babies, it is normal to have some anxiety and reservations about giving consent because you do not know what is going to happen next. It is the cranial therapist's job to explain what they do and allay your concerns. Rest assured that cranial therapy is a safe and gentle therapy; your baby is in good hands. It is important that you are comfortable with this situation.

MOVING INTO TREATMENT AND ESTABLISHING A PRIORITY
The treatment process naturally progresses from the assessment. The cranial therapist will already have a sense

TAKING YOUR BABY TO A CRANIAL THERAPIST

of what needs to happen next and where and how to begin.

The cranial therapist decides which hand hold to use with your baby to begin the treatment. A hand hold is where the therapist places his/her hand, or hands, on your baby. This could be on an arm or leg, their back, pelvis, abdomen or head. Classically they begin by holding one or both feet or legs, or by placing a hand on their back or on their sacrum (the bone at the back of their pelvis). These holds exert no pressure, cause no pain and use the listening touch. The cranial therapist can evaluate your baby's body where their hands are making contact and they can also get a sense of the rest of their body and their state of wholeness.

Remaining neutral, and with the listening touch, the cranial therapist's perceptive sense merges with your baby and their body. After a while, 'something begins to happen' as your baby's body drops into their recovery response. The cranial therapist remains neutral to this and observes and follows what unfolds next. They are a catalyst only: it is your baby's body that is unconsciously in control of this process as they strive for integration, wholeness and balance.

The initial phase of the treatment is often a settling. Babies often present with a sense of being busy, stressed and disorientated. As the cranial therapist continues with their neutral listening touch, this unsettledness begins to calm down. Your baby may be seen to relax.

As they continue to calm, a sense of 'priority' may arise. A priority is the main thing that is going on with your baby right now and what they need help with. Classically this is a mechanical strain, stress response or a state of anger, grief or trauma. However, sometimes the priority is that your baby just needs to be held and supported. When a priority has established, your baby enters the treatment phase.

THIS IS WHAT HAPPENS DURING A TREATMENT

How the cranial therapist manages the treatment phase will depend on how settled or upset your baby is, and what priority has arisen from the assessment. They may continue with the same hand hold, or decide to move to a more appropriate position and hold. The following are the most common priorities.

HELD GRIEF OR ANGER
Many babies hold a priority of grief. Grief indicates that they have not yet got over something upsetting that they have experienced. This is usually their birth, but

could be from being separated from their mother, baby surgery, or time spent in an incubator.

Held grief is stuck emotion. To the cranial therapist it feels like an overwhelming sense of held-back tears, the tears that were never shed. This grief affects the baby's whole body, but is most often felt in the chest and lungs.

As soon as held grief is sensed, it naturally begins to process, it wants to release. As the grief releases its hold, the cranial therapist may feel a softening within the baby. The felt sense of tears becomes a sense of gentle sobbing and then peace. If the baby has been crying excessively, their cry may change to one of feeling sorry for him/herself; sleep may follow. The baby may remain rested for a while. This may be enough for one treatment, or the baby's body may then show another priority and the treatment continues.

The release of anger is similar, but often more dramatic. If the baby is holding a deep sense of anger and the cranial therapist's listening touch perceives this, the anger may begin to surface. As it does so, the baby is likely to cry, increasing in intensity until it becomes an obviously angry cry. They may even go ballistic. This can be deeply upsetting to watch, but it is only the baby putting his/her voice to the held anger within their body. As the anger expresses the baby usually begins to calm down and he/she may suddenly shift into being OK again; sometimes they enter sleep. If anger releases well, it is gone; that angry cry may not occur again.

PROCESSING AND INTEGRATING MECHANICAL STRAINS

Babies, who cry excessively or scream, and who have had a natural delivery or emergency caesarean are likely to have held patterns of compression or mechanical strain in their head and/or body. When such a baby is assessed, it may be clear to the cranial therapist how these strains have been caused, where in the body they are located and what tissues are involved.

For example, a compressional strain may be sensed about the baby's head and involve the cranial bones, the dural membrane, the brain, CSF (cerebrospinal fluid), and the upper neck. It may be clear that the compression occurred during labour.

Mechanical strains and compression resolve in either of two ways. They are sensed as releasing or unwinding.

1. **RELEASING.** From a listening hand hold on the baby's body, the therapist may become aware that the baby's head and neck are compressed. Maintaining the listening and neutral touch engages the baby's recovery system and his/

TAKING YOUR BABY TO A CRANIAL THERAPIST

her body automatically begins to process and integrate the compression. The therapist will feel the compressed pattern begin to shift, then lift. The baby's head will feel softer and cranial-sacral motion returns. The held compression is a physical tension that releases. As this happens the baby remains still and may be observed to relax and even drop off to sleep. Some cranial therapists may change position to hold the baby's head to help complete this decompression.

2. **UNWINDING.** From a hand hold with the baby's head, the cranial therapist's listening touch engages with a twisting strain through their neck and left shoulder. This triggers the recovery system and the baby's body begins to process the strain. This time, however, their body goes into 'unwinding'. The baby's neck, spine and shoulder physically begin to untwist, arch and rotate as his/her body re-experiences and releases this strain from birth. The tissue memory is finding its way out by moving the body into the position necessary for release. The therapist follows these movements with their hands. As you watch, your baby may be twisting around, curling up, or turning over; it can be like they are following their birth pattern and are being reborn. The baby may cry and get upset temporarily as their body processes. As the strain integrates and

resolves, the baby's neck and shoulder relax and he/she calms down and settles. This may be enough for one session, or a second priority may then arise.

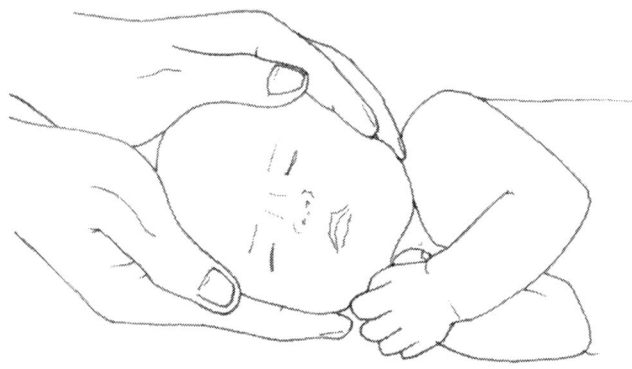

Figure 5. An example of a hand hold on a baby's head. No pressure is used with the listening touch and so the hand hold is not painful.

Different priorities come and go as the baby's body clears itself of its past physical experiences. Over a series of treatment sessions, wholeness, calmness and healthy cranial-sacral motion are restored.

RELEASE OF THE STRESS RESPONSE
When a baby has an active stress response, they are in the fight or flight mode of the sympathetic nervous

system. They may be crying excessively, tense, comfort-feeding, sleeping badly, have digestive issues and be hyper-vigilant, unable to switch off. Cranial therapy helps a stressed baby by calming down the stress response and encouraging the resting mode of the parasympathetic nervous system.

During a treatment, if the cranial therapist engages with a priority of the stress response with their listening touch, they remain neutral and wait and observe. Whatever hand hold is being used, the baby's body will automatically begin to respond. Initially the baby may become more agitated as the stress heightens, then it subsides as his/her body begins the process of stress release. The baby calms from the inside out. They can be seen to slow down, soften, stop crying and sleep; it is as if a cloud of tension has lifted.

As the baby's body relaxes, the cranial therapist will sense cranial-sacral motion dropping from the fast tide to the slow tide, the deeper resting state. Several waves of stress release may occur in one treatment; each time the baby's body relaxes more.

HELPING A BABY THROUGH TRAUMA
Helping a traumatised baby is a different process, requires particular skills and takes time. Trauma is not something a therapist can just fix.

A cranial therapist helps the traumatised baby by creating a safe space for them to re-establish a healthy connection with their body.

A traumatised baby may not be fully present in his/her body and may not wish to be. For them, their body is the vehicle of painful memory. However, unless the baby re-establishes a healthy relationship with their body, they will not fully come out of trauma. It is not possible for anyone to have health unless they are in a good relationship with their body. Again this is achieved through the listening touch of the cranial therapist. The most neutral place on a baby's body is the feet and legs. The cranial therapist takes a gentle hold on their feet and tunes in to their whole body.

If a priority of trauma arises, this comes into the perceptive awareness of the cranial therapist. They can sense that something unpleasant has happened, that the baby is having difficulty with this and that they are not fully engaged with their body. The cranial therapist remains listening and neutral and offers a sense of safety and support to the baby's body through the sense of touch. They can also encourage a deepening into the slow and long tides of cranial-sacral motion.

At some point, the baby's body begins to experience the felt sense of safety encouraged by the listening touch of the cranial therapist; that there is no threat. Gradually the consciousness of the baby begins to connect more with their body. Little by little, the safe and supportive touch creates the sensation of ease, security and eventually pleasure. This floods the baby's brainstem with pleasant sensation and these waves begin to override the painful sensations of their traumatic past experience. The imprint of trauma on the young baby's mind and central nervous system begins to loosen its grip.

As the baby comes into greater relationship with his/her body, any unresolved stress responses held as tissue memory may temporarily trigger and then release. Other priorities of mechanical strain, compression and anger may also arise, process and integrate. This process may take many sessions. Eventually as the felt sense of safety and ease becomes their dominant experience, the baby drops into the slow tides of cranial-sacral motion and their resting state. Peace follows.

WHAT TO EXPECT AFTER A TREATMENT

IMMEDIATE EFFECTS OF CRANIAL THERAPY
Most babies are tired after their first cranial therapy treatment because their body has been processing. If a baby settled well and went off to sleep during treatment, they may continue asleep. Others fall asleep soon after. Some

babies will sleep for an extended period as a catch-up sleep. When a baby wakes up from his/her sleep, their symptoms may be improved or remain unchanged. If nothing has changed, a course of treatment is more likely to help. Excessively crying, screaming and hyper-vigilant babies may not fall asleep during the first few treatments. It is not necessary that a baby falls asleep.

Having a cranial-therapy treatment can make a baby hungry, even if he/she has only recently been fed. They may need a feed immediately afterwards. Feeding after a treatment also helps with settling.

It is not unusual for a baby to cry while receiving cranial therapy; babies do not hold back. This is often a part of their processing. A baby may be finding his/her voice, they may be expressing the emotion of their past experience, or commonly, they are just over-tired and struggling to let go to sleep.

As the baby's mother, it is normal to feel uncomfortable if your baby cries during treatment and occasionally this can become stressful. Speak with the cranial therapist if this happens and you are concerned. As your baby calms and relaxes, the crying stops.

The effect of cranial therapy on a baby does not finish when the therapist has stopped working. Indeed the treatment will work through your baby's body over a period of two to five days. For this reason, never judge the effectiveness of a cranial treatment just on how your baby is immediately afterwards; allow five days.

Some babies show signs of improvement after one session, some are transformed, but please don't expect this. It all depends on what they have been through and how quickly their body responds. If your baby is very unsettled, cries excessively or screams, it may take a series of treatment to make a difference.

If you have any concerns about your baby after a treatment, telephone the cranial therapist concerned – this is part of their service.

WHY SOME BABIES ARE TEMPORARILY WORSE
Although many babies show signs of improvement after their first treatment, a few become temporarily worse. There are three main reasons for this and it is important for the cranial therapist to distinguish the difference between them. These are:

1. A healing reaction
2. An aggravation
3. Coming out of trauma

A healing reaction can cause crying and upset and happens because your baby's body continues to process the effects of the treatment for hours and days afterwards. This is normal and is unlikely to continue for more than one to three days. You can tell if this was a healing reaction because your baby improves as the reaction diminishes. If your baby continues to be very upset for more than three days, it is likely to be an aggravation.

An aggravation may occur if your baby becomes overwhelmed during cranial therapy. If this happens, they begin to cry or scream inconsolably and may fail to stop when the treatment has finished. This reflex reaction may then continue for days. An aggravation may occur if a baby is hypersensitive, but could also be triggered by an over-zealous cranial therapist. It takes a high degree of skill to be able to work with a stressed or traumatised baby without them triggering into overwhelm.

If an aggravation occurs you must telephone the cranial therapist and let them know. They are likely to recommend you and your baby return sooner for a follow-up session. A second treatment usually resolves this.

A traumatised baby may not know what is going on in their body; they became detached from their intolerable birth situation in order to cope. As the baby comes out of trauma and reconnects with his/her body, they become aware of their birth experience and this may trigger their stress response, causing excessive and inconsolable crying. Sometimes this is unavoidable. Cranial therapy is then focused on helping to calm the stress response. These are the babies who may have been unusually quiet since birth and then become very animated when treated. As the course of treatment progresses they calm deeply.

If you have any concerns about how your baby is after cranial therapy it is most important that you speak with the cranial therapist. You may only need reassurance, but there are occasions, as with an aggravation, when the cranial therapist may advise you to return sooner. Good communication is essential.

FOLLOW-UP APPOINTMENTS
Cranial therapy is a process and takes time. Generally, the more treatments your baby has, the more likely he/she is to improve. As treatment progresses you may notice that your child cries or screams less intensely, less often, or not at all. They may sleep better at night and during the day and become able to get themselves off to sleep. They may feed, swallow and breathe more easily. They may be more settled and content. They may smile more, be more social and affectionate. His/her body may feel softer, they may stop wriggling and

arching and be able to lie on their back. Digestive issues such as trapped wind, constipation and straining can improve. Your baby may become totally transformed and become a joy.

Most babies need follow-up appointments and all babies will benefit. Even if your baby is better after one session, it is always advisable to have a check-up. After the first treatment the cranial therapist will have an idea about how many times you will need to return with your baby and when.

Having one treatment per week for three weeks is normal. The cranial therapist may then recommend a few more treatments longer apart – it all depends on progress. A baby will commonly fit into one of the following schedules depending on how they are, who they are and what happened:

1. Having one to three treatments
2. Having five to six treatments
3. Having eight to 10 treatments

If your baby is desperately unsettled with excessive crying or screaming and with a history of a difficult birth, postnatal complications, separation, baby surgery, or prematurity, coming once a week for several weeks is advisable until he/she begins to settle better.

Treatments are then spaced out. This could take more than 10 sessions over several months.

If a baby has an ongoing health issue that is not resolvable, he/she may benefit from regular maintenance treatment. This could be anything from two to 12 times per year.

PRESENCE
A baby who is still experiencing effects from their birth is absorbed by their past. This means their focus in life is on what went before and not on what is happening now: they are not in the present moment.

As cranial therapy begins to work, babies process and integrate the effects of mechanical birth strains, release the stress response, come out of trauma and return to wholeness. Their body becomes physically freer and able to express a slower, more rhythmic pattern of cranial-sacral motion and their focus in life shifts to what is occurring now. This will show as good eye contact, socialisation and affection, improved behaviour and increased interest in their surroundings: the baby becomes totally absorbed by the present moment.

A baby now present and relaxed in his/her body may moan or cry when hungry but is easily satisfied when fed; babies rub their eyes as they become tired and then drift off to sleep; they smile and laugh when happy or amused; they will watch and attempt to interact with all that goes on around them. Now their past experience is but a distant tissue memory – they are able to get on with their life and you are able to enjoy being his/her parent.

Chapter 7

ADAPTATION TO BIRTH

Today, only the minority of babies born receive cranial therapy. This is because it is a relatively new therapy; most people and most parents either don't know about it or do not understand it. It is not recognised by governments or health authorities, and availability of cranial therapists in some countries is poor, if it exists at all, but the tide is turning.

If your baby cries excessively or screams, you may have been told they will grow out of it. This is true in most cases, but there is a cost. This chapter discusses what happens to birth strains, stresses and trauma if they remain in your baby's body and what the consequences may be as he/she develops into an infant, child and adult. What happens as your baby moves away from their birth and prenatal experience and into present time is then considered.

LIFE IS OFTEN ABOUT ADAPTATION

THE ADAPTATION RESPONSE
Human beings have evolved a further survival response. As well as the stress response, the trauma response and the recovery response, there is also the adaptation response.

When we are affected by something relatively minor, such as a cold, cut, strain, emotional upset, or an easy birth, our body gets over it and makes a full recovery. Anything more serious may leave its mark. If something major happens to us, like a severe accident or injury, a major operation, a huge emotional shock, a mental breakdown, or a difficult birth, our body may not be able to get over it well. To ensure that we are able to carry on our body adapts.

Adaptation means that our body and mind repair sufficiently well in order for us to carry on living, but essentially we are patched together. From then onwards we hold physical, emotional and mental scars. These scars may affect our health, our resilience and our confidence.

ADAPTATION TO BIRTH

Adaptation is not ideal because it becomes a long-term response. The wisdom of the body says that right now I am unable to deal with this situation completely, so I will do whatever is necessary in order to carry on. At a future date, when life becomes more safe and settled, I will re-visit what happened and complete the healing process. For many of us this never happens; our wounds remain locked away as tissue memory within the structure of our body and within our mind. We carry them for the rest of our lives. The same is true for babies.

It is the power of the adaptation response and the ability to carry on that is so remarkable with human beings. Many people, including babies and children, are able to carry on after the most difficult experiences, life-threatening situations and injuries, and live a rewarding life.

HOW ADAPTATION AFFECTS HEALTH
The effect of an adapted state on the human body is tissue contraction. As our body repairs and heals physically, emotionally and mentally, our tissues tighten up and contract.

A cut heals by forming scar tissue. The scar tissue is thicker and more contracted than the original skin and can tighten, causing a distortion. Similarly, bone fractures heal with a callus – they form a bony lump.

The mended fracture site is thicker, tighter and stronger than the original bone.

If we have adapted to an emotional shock, we continue to hold that emotional tension within the structure of our body as tissue memory, often within our organs. We may hold patterns of sadness, grief or anger. This held emotion becomes a physical tension, creating tissue contraction.

We also adapt to mental trauma. When events unfold that our minds are unable to tolerate or integrate, thoughts and memories get sealed off in our body. They are hidden out of the way in the hope that they will be forgotten. It is often within the structure of the brain that the held thought patterns create tissue contraction. These patterns of brain contraction affect our mind and may haunt us unconsciously, affecting our behaviour, thinking processes and dreams. They may cause us to become withdrawn, anxious, fearful, even depressed.

Health is about freedom. The freedom of blood and fluids to circulate into and out of our cells and tissues; the freedom of transmission of nerve impulses; the freedom of movement; the freedom of creativity, the freedom of self-expression and the freedom of cranial-sacral motion. Anything that restricts freedom affects health. Tissue contraction in areas of the body affected by adaptation to physical, emotional or mental events restricts freedom and sooner or later symptom patterns arise, sometimes disease. Restoring freedom leads to health; cranial therapy helps to restore tissue freedom.

GAINING MORE CLARITY
An important part of cranial therapy training is that the students have regular cranial therapy treatments from an experienced practitioner during their study. Frequently they carry on this practice throughout their working lives.

The reason for this is twofold. By being a client yourself you become familiar with the clinical setting and how different therapists work. Also, by receiving cranial therapy, you gain deeper insight into yourself, your body, your past and your state of health: you gain more clarity.

During the sequence of treatments the student cranial therapist gets to know his/her own living anatomy and how it functions. Students experience at first hand their own states of adaptation (we all have these) and how they process and integrate. Cranial therapists who work with babies and children will have re-experienced and integrated aspects of their own childhood and their birth process.

Therapeutically working through and finding peace with his/her own history allows a cranial therapist to be more available and receptive to the needs of others. If you have more clarity in your own body, you have greater empathy and compassion and are in a better position to resonate with whatever someone else has experienced. This helps cranial therapists with their ability to assess and treat their clients.

PRENATAL INFLUENCES
A further reason why some babies may not have responded well to cranial therapy is because the cause of their symptoms could lie in the prenatal period. The prenatal period is the time between conception and birth.

To complete the understanding of crying babies and birth, the time a baby spends within his/her mother's reproductive system must be considered. After all, nine months of gestation is a pretty long time to be hanging out in an enclosed space and within someone else's body.

Much happens during pregnancy. The mother's body goes through physiological changes and both parents need to adjust their lives for the arrival of their child. Unexpected events also occur, such as the loss of a job, having to move house, illness or bereavement. Any or all of these effects could be an influence on the developing baby, who remains constantly present and aware.

ADAPTATION TO BIRTH

Prenatal work is a specialised area of cranial therapy. To become familiar with this requires post-graduate training. Not all cranial therapists who work with babies are trained and experienced in prenatal therapy and so they may not yet be able to perceive prenatal influences. This is OK because the main issues facing most excessively crying or screaming babies are the effects from labour, delivery and the postnatal period.

For a cranial therapist to develop the necessary skills to work with prenatal influences he/she studies embryology (the science of how the body forms from the fertilised egg into a foetus) and foetal development. They also need to continue to receive cranial therapy, but from a cranial therapist experienced in prenatal work. This enables the cranial therapist to deepen his/her understanding of their living anatomy and to help integrate their own embryological experiences. The knowledge of our prenatal life from conception to birth is held within our body and cells too, as tissue memory.

ADAPTATION IN BABIES

BABIES ADAPT TO THEIR EXPERIENCE
A baby who has had a straightforward natural birth and an easy postnatal period will usually settle well within a few weeks. Their body adjusts and rebalances to life outside the womb and they are able to get on with life.

They still have needs, but they won't be crying excessively or screaming.

A baby more affected by his/her birth may be a little unsettled and upset but they are essentially OK, and with love and support, move on and enjoy their babyhood. A couple of cranial therapy treatments will help release any minor strains and stresses and aid the settling process.

It is these babies who experience a more difficult birth, or postnatal complications, who are unable to just get on. They are the ones who are likely to be very unsettled, cry excessively, or scream. Such babies may be in ongoing pain, holding compression or mechanical strains, have an active stress response or they may be holding a deep sense of trauma. Getting on in life is a struggle. These babies have to adapt to what they have experienced because their body is unable to get over what happened. As time goes by, they settle into their adaptations. The excessive crying and screaming eventually stop, but may be replaced by other functional and behavioural issues.

Adaptation means that the mechanical strains of labour and birth do not just disappear; they may modify but largely remain held within the baby's body as patterns of tissue compression and tightness: the stress response does not just stop, it persists. The baby remains reactive and in a heightened state of alertness, unable to let go

ADAPTATION TO BIRTH

into their natural resting state. Trauma does not go away either; it gets shut off deep within the baby's body and subconscious mind, and their behaviour will reflect this. Many babies adapt to their previous experiences; these shape their life and are reflected in their symptom patterns.

ADAPTATION TO STRAINS AND STRESSES

If a baby is holding a birth pattern of mechanical compression or tissue strain this just does not disappear as they grow. The compression and tightness in their tissues remains and it will stay throughout life as tissue memory unless it is released by a therapeutic process, such as cranial therapy.

In a baby this may show as a tight and fidgety body. Such babies are not easy to cuddle because they are constantly on the move and they do not soften when held. Other indications of adaptations to mechanical strain in babies include: having a distortion in the shape of their skull, ongoing difficulty in turning the neck in one or both directions, arching of the neck, arching of the whole spine, having trouble lying on their back, being unable to lie straight and digestive or breathing issues resulting from disturbance of the cranial nerve called the vagus nerve (refer back to the cranial nerves and figure 3. in chapter 3).

It is the same with stress patterns. If a baby becomes very stressed during birth, the stress will remain in his/her body tissues and nervous system, often creating a condition of over-alertness, hyper-vigilance and trouble letting go. It can result in poor sleep, feeding issues, digestive disturbances, irregular breathing, baby asthma and irritability. This tendency may continue as the baby grows and may impact into childhood and even adulthood.

If a baby is holding an adapted pattern to stress, his/her resilience to stressful experiences at a later age will be reduced. If your body and brain are already tense, there is nowhere for new stresses to go. That is why babies already stressed from their birth have more trouble coping with the additional stress of teething.

With many children and teenagers their first real stress is with school exams. Typically, a teenager who fails to cope well with exam pressure will already be holding a stress pattern, often from his/her birth or postnatal period. A baby treated with cranial therapy is calmer and reacts better to stressful situations. This is because their relaxed body is more capable of absorbing the stresses of life without immediately going into overwhelm.

ADAPTATION AND TRAUMA
If a baby has had a traumatic experience during or

after birth, he/she adapts to what happened. How they adapt often depends on their strength of character. If they are a fighter, they can be successful in overcoming any adversity but if they are more of a victim then they may continue to struggle, lack confidence and be withdrawn.

Babies suffering from trauma may continue to cry excessively and scream throughout their babyhood and into infancy. They may continue to have issues with their digestion and to have problems with sleep and letting go to sleep, both day and night. A traumatised baby may not be much fun; they can be sad and grumpy, slow to smile. Some are more insular, undemonstrative and have poor social engagement; others want to be held constantly.

Most premature babies have an adapted state to trauma. As they grow they may begin to show evidence of sensory processing issues, poor concentration, slow learning and delayed development. They may be prone to angry tantrums, obsessive behaviours and easily become overwhelmed. If your baby is showing these tendencies, he/she may need additional support from health services. Cranial therapy can help too. The gentle, listening touch of the cranial therapist establishes a safe level of contact with your baby's body and it is this that can help lead them gradually out of the trauma response and to begin to establish a healthier re-engagement with life. It is not possible to recover from trauma without help.

CRANIAL THERAPY AND ADAPTATION

The cranial therapy treatment of states of adaptation in babies and infants is more complex. There are two reasons for this:

1. **Familiarity.** The human body becomes familiar with, and learns to accept its adaptations; they become friends. The body may not wish to give up something that it knows and once served a useful purpose - the ability to carry on. It's like saying goodbye to an old friend. We are like this as adults: it is easier to carry on a behavioural pattern that no longer serves us than to dare to change.
2. **Fear of the unknown.** If the human body is given the opportunity to embrace a new and healthier way of being, often it will reject it. Our primitive nervous system is primed to believe any alternative is a threat and may make life worse (better the devil you know). Some adults unconsciously do this during a course of therapy; they decide to stop coming right at the point of change. This is called resistance.

Sometimes during the treatment of a baby a held state of adaptation begins to process. The baby may be easier for several days and then the same symptoms return: their body decided to revert back to the original adaptation. It may then take several sessions for the adapted pattern to process well enough to release and integrate.

The key to this issue with cranial therapy is safety and perseverance. If the baby's body begins to experience the pleasant sensation of the listening touch as unthreatening, their body begins to relax. The wisdom of the body realises there is a healthier option than the state of adaptation and embraces the greater sense of ease and freedom. This process may take time and is one reason why the treatment process may take five or six sessions, or more.

ADAPTATIONS IN CHILDREN

Cranial therapy is not just a treatment for babies; children and adults benefit too. Whatever complaint a child has, it is common for the child's body to bring up a birth issue as a priority within the first three treatments, sometimes the first one. This is because birth is often the most significant event so far in a young child's life and adaptations from birth have a big effect on them and their health.

ASTHMA

Asthma can be caused by an activated stress response that overstimulates the lungs and respiratory system, resulting in hypersensitivity. This often relates to a previous stressful experience or injury, which in asthmatic babies and young children is frequently their birth.

Case study 6: *Jack is only three years old. He was diagnosed with asthma at the age of 18 months, takes a steroid inhaler twice daily and has been hospitalised on three occasions.*

Assessing Jack while he was sitting on his mother's lap revealed the following: deep distress in his body, as if he had failed to cope with something that had happened; a panic reaction in his lungs and diaphragm and a held sense of stress and panic in his cranial dura (the lining of the brain).

My understanding was that Jack had experienced his birth as out of control. His head had been severely strained, which had triggered a tissue panic reaction in his dural membranes, lungs and diaphragm. His lungs remained stressed and hyper-reactive, predisposing him to asthmatic episodes. Jack's mother confirmed there were complications with his birth. He was born by elective caesarean section, but had to be extracted by ventouse!

The first cranial therapy session released the panic and distress in Jack's body, lungs, diaphragm and cranial dural membranes. After this he was able to reduce his inhaler to once daily. After three treatments he no longer needed his inhalers. Two years later and he is still off his inhalers and has not returned to hospital. His mother reports that he has not suffered from hayfever since.

ADAPTATION TO BIRTH

GLUE EAR
The bones that form the sides of our skull are called the temporal bones and they house our hearing mechanism. The prominence of the temporal bones means that they are often compressed during birth and can twist so one side of the head becomes more forward than the other.

The middle ear is an air-filled space within each temporal bone and contains three little bones called the ossicles, which conduct the sound waves from the eardrum to the brain. Children are diagnosed with glue ear if they have an active infection, or fluid, in their middle ear. This can cause pressure, pain and congestion, resulting in hearing loss.

Case study 7: *Tom is five years old. He had had hearing loss over a period of two years and had been diagnosed with glue ear. His mother was recommended to try cranial therapy by a friend.*

My initial assessment of Tom using the listening touch revealed that he was holding a deeply-held grief pattern. His nervous system was in a state of activation, as were his ears and eyes. The base of his skull and temporal bones were holding a compressive strain; he had tension in his jaw and throat. His ears felt congested, as though they needed to 'breathe'.

My conclusion was that the base and sides of Tom's skull were compressed during his birth and this remained as a mechanical adaptation. His held grief, nervous system activation and sensory activation were caused by a trauma he had not yet got over. The restriction in Tom's

> *temporal bones, jaw and throat were preventing normal fluid drainage, leading to the congestion in his middle ears. Tom's mum explained that he had had a difficult birth and stomach surgery as a baby; the surgery was the cause of his trauma.*
>
> *During his first treatment the pattern of held grief released and the activation in his nervous system and sensory system began to settle. After three cranial therapy sessions Tom's mother reported that he was hearing better and a subsequent full range of hearing tests at the hospital were normal. Reassessing Tom showed that the base of his skull, his temporal bones, jaw and throat were free of compression and moving freely – the congestion in his ears had cleared.*

NIGHT TERRORS

Night terrors cause a child or baby to suddenly start crying severely or screaming in their sleep and may involve thrashing around or sleep walking. They are not awake.

The most common cause of night terrors is previous trauma – the adapted trauma response surfaces from the unconscious mind while the child is sleeping and actively affects his/her dream state. With children and babies the cause is commonly unresolved trauma from their birth, or surgery.

> **Case study 8:** *Oliver is eight years old and has suffered from night terrors for five years. Initially he would cry and scream in his sleep, but this progressed to restlessness, shouting and sometimes sleep walking. During the day he can be easily distracted, angry and out of control.*
>
> *The cranial therapy assessment revealed an unconsciously held trauma pattern in Oliver's chest and brain stem. He had anger held in the left side of his brain and left eye and his dural membranes were tightly held, with no clear cranial-sacral motion. Oliver was born by elective caesarean section, but he had had abdominal surgery as a baby. His surgery was the most likely cause of his trauma pattern and anger.*
>
> *During his three cranial therapy sessions Oliver's body released its tightness and held anger and cranial-sacral motion returned to his body and nervous system. His unconscious trauma adaptation processed and integrated. Oliver was now sleeping soundly, had had no further night terrors and was calmer during the day.*

SOCIALISATION AND BEHAVIOUR

Learning, processing, socialisation and behavioural problems are not uncommon in children. Although they can have other causes, the nature of the child's birth and how he/she has adapted to it are big factors. Ideally the assessment and treatment of any child with learning or behavioural difficulties should involve cranial therapy. This is to rule out adaptations from birth as a causative or aggravating factor and to treat them if present.

> **Case study 9:** *Rebecca's mother explained that her six-year-old daughter finds life hard; she struggles, worries and is anxious. She is not very affectionate, has difficulty relating to her peers and spends much time on her own. Rebecca is over-sensitive, obsessive, cannot cope with chaos and can get angry.*
>
> *Assessing Rebecca showed that her central nervous system was in a state of hyper-arousal with rapid cranial-sacral motion. She had a marked twisting of her sphenoid bone (which forms part of the base of the skull) and poor sensory processing. Rebecca's brain was very tense and it felt as though her mind had withdrawn deep within itself. Her mother described the long and difficult birth, with Rebecca becoming stuck during delivery.*
>
> *Rebecca is a naturally hypersensitive child. During birth she went into the trauma mode as she was no longer able to cope with her experience. She withdrew deep within herself and became socially disengaged. This remained as an adapted state. Sphenoid bone strain interferes with normal sensory processing, explaining why Rebecca quickly becomes overwhelmed when too much is going on. She is unable to help how she is.*
>
> *With three craniosacral therapy sessions the stress in Rebecca's central nervous system released, cranial-sacral motion slowed down, her brain softened and her mind expanded into it. Her sphenoid bone rebalanced, allowing her brain to process more effectively. Rebecca's mother reported that her daughter is now a happy and affectionate child. She is able to relate to her family and her peers and is no longer aggressive. Her school have noticed her transformation too.*

Having a broader understanding of the human body, living anatomy, cranial-sacral motion and birth adaptations gives valuable insights into the health and diagnosis of our children. Cranial therapy provides an additional, gentle and drug-free way of helping them.

ADAPTATION IN ADULTS AND MOVING INTO PRESENT TIME

It is amazing how many health issues in adults have their roots in adapted patterns from their birth. This applies to both physical and mental health complaints.

REACTIVATION OF OLD WOUNDS
Many interesting phenomena arise in the world of cranial therapy. One of these is the re-activation of old wounds. An old wound is an injury the body has previously sustained and had to adapt to because it was unable to recover completely at the time. The injury remains dormant as tissue memory. Later in life, if the same part of the body is injured again, the original injury re-surfaces. The present injury will then only resolve properly if the original injury integrates too. This phenomenon explains why some people fail to get over recent injuries – there are deeper layers to address.

Case study 10: John, aged 37, strained his right forearm and injured his lower back playing golf. He complained of a dull ache in his lower back, sciatic pain in his right buttock and arm pain when using his right hand. John failed to respond to physiotherapy and osteopathic manipulation had only made his back worse.

> *Assessing John revealed he had a twisted sacrum, compressed lower back and a twisting pattern through his spine and upper neck. The base of his skull and right shoulder were compressed too. This was causing muscle tension through his arm.*
>
> *Within minutes of his first treatment John's body revealed a birth pattern and went into tissue release. His head, neck, spine and sacrum had become very compressed and twisted during his passage through the birth canal. After birth, his body had adapted to this pattern and this adaptation had remained dormant and symptomless until now: his golfing strain had re-activated it.*
>
> *John did not know anything about his birth, so he asked his mother. She told him it had been a long labour and difficult second stage as his right shoulder had become stuck.*
>
> *After one treatment John reported his buttock and right arm were free of pain and his lower back was much better. After three sessions, he was out of pain and back playing golf. The release and integration of his birth pattern enabled his body to quickly recover from the recent strain.*

MENTAL HEALTH

In the world of health and the human body everything that affects the body affects the mind and everything that affects the mind affects the body. For example, if you think of something unpleasant your heart will feel heavy and your shoulders collapse. Smile and you will automatically sit upright and feel more optimistic.

Mental health disorders are not just problems of the

mind; they involve the body too. The majority of people with mental health issues have a history of trauma, whether from accidents, injuries, or abuse.

There are regular findings when a cranial therapist assesses a client with depression following a head injury. These are a compressive strain of the head, dural membranes and the brain. To a cranial therapist, a compressed brain feels heavy, dark and squashed and may express no cranial-sacral motion. When the brain is compressed the clarity of mind and thoughts are affected too. These changes can be perceived with the listening touch.

If your head and brain are in an adapted state of compression, it can feel as though you are trapped in your head. You may feel cut off, distant and lack space. This can affect your mood and how and what you think. Your thoughts may become darker and more pessimistic as your relationship with the world shrinks.

Case study 11: *Julie has a long history of depression. She complains of feeling constantly tired, permanently worried and has dark thoughts.*

The listening touch of the cranial therapist reveals that Julie's skull is tight and compressed, as if there is no space for her brain. Her brain feels as though it is being crushed by pressure. This is a compressive pattern from birth.

> *During her first treatment Julie's cranial bones and dural membranes released, the state of compression lifted and her brain began to feel more expansive and express cranial-sacral motion. She entered a deep state of relaxation. Attending her second session, Julie reported that a 'dark cloud had lifted' and she now feels calmer, brighter and happier. Her friends have noticed this too.*

A BIT MORE HISTORY

Psycho-analysis, developed by medical doctor and psychiatrist Sigmund Freud (1856–1939), changed the understanding of mental health in the 19th and 20th centuries and the treatment approaches to it. He established the idea that how we have adapted to previous difficult events in our lives affects our mental health now, and that in becoming conscious of these old, painful memories, our thinking and behaviour changes in the present.

Although some people benefited from psychoanalysis, spending many years of one's life in weekly therapy was beyond most people's motivation and means, and the therapeutic value of psychoanalysis has always been questioned.

It was later that Wilhelm Reich (1897–1957), a pupil of Dr Freud, further revolutionised the understanding of mental health with his theory of body armouring. He realised that we hold past memories and traumas within our body structure (tissue memory), creating holding patterns, or armouring. It was this shift into acknowledging that body and mind are intrinsically linked that triggered a wave of new body/mind therapies in the 1960s and 70s. These included primal therapy, bio-energetic therapy, rebirthing, gestalt therapy and rolfing.

Osteopath Dr John Upledger was influenced by this growing human potential movement and he embraced the new body/mind understanding. This inspired his move away from the classical practice of cranial osteopathy and into developing the new field of craniosacral therapy.

Craniosacral therapy and cranial osteopathy have continued to evolve. The understanding of cranial-sacral motion has reached a greater sense of completion by embracing the state of oneness of our living anatomy with the rhythms and tides of the essence of life.

MOVING INTO PRESENT TIME
When a cranial therapist is treating a baby, child or an adult, the priorities that first arise are almost always those associated with past events. This shows that the human body adapts to what has happened and stores this information as tissue memory. Accessing tissue memory tells the story of our past.

Unfortunately, it is the unpleasant, stressful and physically or mentally traumatic events that get stored because it is these events that overwhelm us and lead to adaptation and contraction within our body. Pleasant and joyous events leave us with great memories and feelings, but not tissue tightness because they do not cause contraction.

Historically it was understood that if we got in touch with, and re-experienced a past memory, then the memory would resolve and disappear, leaving us free from our past. This has proved not to be the case. It is possible to become stuck in repetitively reliving patterns from the past, thinking we are changing but actually going nowhere. Something more needs to happen for the healing process to complete.

Therapeutically, it has become important to relate to the past from a new angle. Past experiences arise as priorities during cranial therapy because they are still active in the present moment: we are living and expressing our past. Unsettled babies are still experiencing the effects of their birth because these effects are active in their body now. Tissue memory is in present time. In reality there is no past. Past is but an impression, an illusion; a dream.

ADAPTATION TO BIRTH

The practice of cranial therapy creates a safe space for enabling a baby, child or adult to become present in their body tissues. If you are present in your body, you know more clearly who you are, and you are living your life as it is unfolding now. This is not always a great experience initially, because you may not like what you see and your present circumstances may be pretty awful, but at least you know where you are at: you are experiencing your truth. Only when you have fully arrived can you move on and this is what babies do.

A cranial therapist working with a baby is present and complete in his/her own body. By remaining neutral and using the listening touch, the baby is able to become present in their body too and the effects of their past may show up as priorities now.

As a baby drops into the slower tides of cranial-sacral motion, the wisdom of their body realises that the patterns of their past, held in their body as tissue memory, are in the way of them fully expressing life as it is occurring now. They have had their use and are no longer needed. As these patterns naturally begin to process and integrate, the baby's body and mind release and become clearer.

Their strains, stresses, trauma patterns and adaptations are the armouring that keeps a baby away from his/her present experience. As the baby experiences the physical sensations of life as safe, pleasurable, interesting and rewarding, there is no further need for armour. Health then follows.

A baby becoming fully present in his/her body holds no contraction. Their whole body is able to freely express cranial-sacral motion – bones, membranes, fasciae, muscles, organs and fluids. They are alive to their experience and their body tissues are expressing this. There is no excessive crying or screaming because they have contentment and peace. The baby is no longer living his/her life from the perspective of their past; they have arrived in present time.

Case study 12: *Felix is one years old. His mother explained that he has been unsettled since birth and he cries inconsolably, screams and has night terrors. She described Felix as never still, difficult to cuddle, frustrated, angry and unhappy. He had a quick natural birth (three hours) without complications, but was born three weeks early.*

Assessing Felix revealed that he was in trauma mode and had severe compression and twisting of his cranial bones, spine and dural membranes, with no evident cranial-sacral motion. These effects were due to the speed of his labour and delivery and because Felix was not ready to be born.

Despite responding well to each session of cranial therapy Felix's symptoms hardly changed until after his fifth session. Since then his mother reports that he has become more communicative; he has started to talk and walk. Felix no longer cries, screams or has nightmares.

ADAPTATION TO BIRTH

He wakes only once at night but goes off to sleep again. In the morning he wakes happy and smiling. Reassessing Felix showed that he is no longer in trauma and that his spine, cranial bones and dural membranes are balanced, free of tightness and expressing cranial-sacral motion.

YOUR NEXT STEP

This is the concluding section. It contains a brief book review, takes you through your next step, provides details of some professional associations of cranial therapists, considers the wider role of cranial therapy in today's society and gives you some background information about the author, Peter Zealley ND, DO, BCST.

THE BOOK REVIEW

Society often portrays pregnancy, giving birth and being a parent as one of the most rewarding and happiest times of life. For some parents this is undoubtedly so, but for others, their experience can be different.

Your pregnancy may have been trying, especially if you felt ill for most of it. Giving birth, especially for the first time, may not have gone according to plan, was far more painful than you ever imagined and may have been a stressful and traumatic experience. There may have been postnatal complications too. If after all that, your baby is unsettled and cries excessively, inconsolably or screams, you may rightfully wonder what happened to the joys of parenthood.

If your friends' babies are happy and content while yours constantly struggles, you may feel even more alone. You are trying to cope in a very difficult circumstance, to which no one has an answer and which can become intolerable. Even help and advice from your doctor, midwife and health visitor may not be enough to change the situation. You continue as best you can because you have to.

The message of this book is simple: those babies who cry and scream excessively and who are otherwise healthy frequently do so because they are still experiencing the effects of their birth. Their little body may be holding and reacting to the compressive and straining forces of the birth process; they may be over-activated by their stress response and some may even be traumatised.

Being able to understand more clearly what your baby is experiencing is the first step on the road towards helping them. Once it is recognised what is troubling them, something more can be done to help.

This is where craniosacral therapists and cranial osteopaths come in; they are the experts in this field. These therapists are professionally trained to sense with their hands the strains, stresses, traumas and emotional upset left behind in the structure of the human body as a result of events that have happened. With babies this is frequently their birth and/or postnatal experience. You have a new possibility for help.

With parental consent, the gentle and safe treatment-approach of cranial therapy can be employed to begin to help your baby's body process, to release and integrate what they have experienced. This allows them to become whole, content and able to participate fully in their life as it is unfolding now.

YOUR NEXT STEP

If you reflect on your process of giving birth and what has happened since then, you may recognise that both you and your baby have been through a lot in a very short space of time.

It is important for you as a mother to acknowledge how you are now, and whether you have recovered sufficiently from your pregnancy and the birth itself. The birth may or may not have gone according to plan and there may have been unforeseen postnatal complications.

YOUR NEXT STEP

You may be stressed or traumatised from the experience and your body may still be physically healing. If your baby cries excessively or screams, you may be exhausted, struggling to cope and not knowing where next to turn. Whatever your experience, it is necessary that you have adequate support from a combination of a partner, family, friends and the medical services, and that where possible, you are living in an environment that is safe and conducive to your well-being and that of your child.

Your main concern now is your baby. As a parent you will become familiar with his/her different cries. If you are experiencing recurrent or ongoing periods of excessive crying and screaming on a daily basis despite meeting all your baby's needs, you will realise that something is not right for them. In this situation you need professional help.

If extreme crying is a sudden change in your baby's behaviour it is initially essential to rule out an acute medical illness. To do this you must consult your doctor and if you are still concerned, seek a second opinion. It is always advisable to consult your doctor in the first instance if you have a concern about your baby.

If your baby is suffering from a regular pattern of excessive crying or screaming, which may be associated with other symptoms such as trapped wind, colic, poor sleep, fractiousness or body arching, he/she may be suffering from the most common cause of excessive crying and screaming in babies. This is that they have not yet got over the experience of their birth.

As you look back on what you and your baby have experienced in your life together so far, you may recognise some stressful or traumatic events that may account for this. However, if you had a good natural delivery or elective caesarean section, these experiences can still upset your baby. Your baby's reaction to birth can depend on their character and how they coped or failed to cope with their experience.

Even if cranial therapy is new to you, you may now have enough knowledge of its theory and practice to be willing to try this treatment approach for your baby. It is gentle and safe and is the most appropriate therapy for unsettled, crying and screaming babies.

Once you have the contact details of a cranial therapist, telephone them. It is often best to speak with the cranial therapist about your baby and your concerns when you make your first appointment. If you get an answerphone, leave them a message; often a busy therapist is not able to answer your call straightaway.

YOUR NEXT STEP

When you begin the treatment with your baby keep an open mind. Cranial therapy is subtle and is a process that takes time: perseverance is the key to a successful outcome. Initially anticipate your baby may need six sessions; they may only need to return once or twice. If that is not enough to make a difference, carry on. The cranial therapist will guide you through the treatment process.

Working with babies is one of the most rewarding and challenging aspects of being a cranial therapist. Cranial therapy is an effective therapy: time and time again it helps babies to stop crying and screaming, it frequently transforms the lives of babies and their families but there may be times when a baby has an underlying health issue and the results are less forthcoming. As professional therapists we strive to gain in knowledge and experience in order to continually improve our skill and effectiveness with the listening touch.

If your baby appears not to be responding to cranial therapy you need to discuss this with the cranial therapist. They may suggest you need to carry on a bit longer, seek a second opinion with a colleague, or to return to your doctor for further help, advice, or referral. It is also worth considering the therapy of homeopathy. This is another natural therapy and often helps babies and children. With the use of natural remedies homeopathy can support the work already done by a cranial therapist and the medical professions.

Your cranial therapist may becomes part of your family health network. They are someone you can turn to at any time for help and advice regarding your own health and the health of your baby as he/she progresses through infancy and childhood. You are likely to return another time with your next baby.

PROFESSIONAL ASSOCIATIONS

All cranial therapists must complete a professional training in order to become accepted as a registered member of a professional cranial association. As part of their membership they have to hold professional indemnity insurance and to continue with their professional development on an annual basis.

In the UK there are three main registers of cranial therapists. These are:

1. The Craniosacral Therapy Association (CSTA) www.craniosacral.co.uk
2. The Upledger Institute UK www.upledger.co.uk
3. The General Osteopathic Council (GOsC) www.osteopathy.org.uk

Countries outside of the UK may have their own craniosacral and osteopathic organisations and registers.

The Upledger Institute is based in America and has branches in many countries.

There is also an international craniosacral therapy organisation: The International Affiliation of Biodynamic Trainings (IABT) found at www.biodynamic-craniosacral.org

THE ROLE FOR CRANIAL THERAPY

Cranial therapy in its different forms is an advancing profession. Each year hundreds of students are trained from the different schools, and cranial therapy training takes place in an increasing number of countries worldwide. Many people have changed their careers to become a cranial therapist. Its popularity is due to the combination of safety, gentleness and effectiveness; cranial therapy frequently makes a difference.

As the majority of births take place in hospital, there is a strong case for making cranial therapy automatically and freely available to babies at their point of entry. Issues related to a baby's birth experience are best resolved as soon as possible. Babies will then settle quicker, feed and sleep better and are less likely to develop health and behavioural issues as they develop and grow. There would be no need for adaptation. Then, not only will the baby enjoy his/her body and their experience of life more completely, family life would be easier too – for all its members.

Any idea of transforming society for the better needs to start at the beginning, that is with conception, prenatal care, babies and birth. If our babies and we ourselves receive the help we need to become free, whole and at peace within our own living anatomy, we will become more compassionate, accepting of differences and present to the challenges of life that face us all.

ABOUT PETER ZEALLEY

I have held a lifelong interest in nature and natural healing. This led me to train at the British College of Naturopathy and Osteopathy in London at the age of 20. After graduation, I set up a private practice in Devon, where I still live today. I am married with three children and so far, one grandchild.

Naturopathy and osteopathy gave me a good understanding of the human body and natural methods of treatment to help people improve their health. My sensitive, perceptive and inquisitive nature then drew me into my own personal journey. I became experientially involved in the human potential movement and then the practices of meditation and natural healing. At the same time, as my awareness unfolded, professionally I moved through the fields of cranial osteopathy, Upledger craniosacral therapy and more recently into biodynamic craniosacral therapy. For me life continues to be a quest of integrating the unseen rhythms and tides of life with the anatomy of our body and mind and in how this experience leads to the greater expression of our unique identity.

Information about my private practice, social media and contact details are available on my website:

www.peterzealley.com

CPSIA information can be obtained at www.ICGtesting.com
Printed in the USA
LVOW10s1925120315

430306LV00028B/1093/P